Diana L. Gustafson, RN, MEd, PhD
Editor

Unbecoming Mothers
The Social Production
of Maternal Absence

Pre-publication
REVIEWS,
COMMENTARIES,
EVALUATIONS . . .

"*Unbecoming Mothers* is an important contribution to the evolving theoretical and experiential literature dealing with the realities of mothering in the twenty-first century. The book disrupts the gendered representations of acceptable parenting behaviors for mothers and fathers and creates room for a rich scope of mothering roles. The book allows maternal absence to be understood from the subjective position of mothers as well as from the viewpoint of the children and other non-mothers. The challenges that each of the chapters levels against conceptions about unbecoming mothers work not only to free those mothers from the social constraints but to free all mothers to mother in the ways that they are able to in the circumstances in which they find themselves. Opening the ways we think about mothers and the mother-work they perform allows us to envision a more tolerant scope for the care and nurture of our children.

Gustafson's collection underlines the impact of the structural factors that shape the ways women carry out their motherwork and undermines the notion that these ways are shaped only by women's contextual, individualistic choices. It also foregrounds the experiences of 'unbecoming mothers' who have not been heard from in the literature thus far. The personhood of mothers is reaffirmed in powerful ways by the variety and diversity of the voices heard in this book."

Lorna Turnbull, LLB, LLM, JSD
Assistant Professor, Faculty of Law,
University of Manitoba, Canada;
Author of *Double Jeopardy:*
Motherwork and the Law

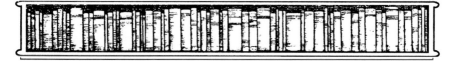

More pre-publication
REVIEWS, COMMENTARIES, EVALUATIONS . . .

"*Unbecoming Mothers* is an important addition to debates on motherhood. Recognizing that mothering is a diverse experience done by both biological and social mothers, this collection focuses on biological mothers' complex experiences of living apart from their children. The chapters range across academic disciplines, including social policy, anthropology, and performing arts, to explore dominant discourses of motherhood in, primarily, Canada, Australia, the United States, and early modern Britain. The result is to highlight motherhood that either deviates from these norms due to being nonresidential or becomes nonresidential due to perceived deviance from these norms.

One of the most valuable aspects of this book is the way it gives voice to women's real experiences of unbecoming motherhood, especially Aboriginal women (in Canada and Australia), young mothers in care, and African-American girls in kinship care, who are less frequently heard."

Jennifer Marchbank, PhD
Senior Lecturer, School of Health and Social Sciences,
Coventry University,
United Kingdom

"*Unbecoming Mothers* is a truly important book. It examines the topic of motherhood from the inside out (the experiences of mothers) and from the outside in (the views of the children who grew up without their mothers). The materials are fascinating, combing historical and contemporary viewpoints as well as experiential and third-person accounts. This book significantly affects the way readers think about motherhood by helping readers understand the reasons that lead to absentee mothering, the silent coercions that lead women to give up their babies for adoption, the pain that children experience when their families do not conform to what is seen as the norm, and the social expectations confronting young mothers in state care that lead, paradoxically, to the opposite effects of those intended. This book should be read by everyone who studies families, parenthood, and gender."

Margrit Eichler, FRSC
Professor, Sociology and Equity Studies in Education,
OISE, University of Toronto,
Canada

The Haworth Clinical Practice Press™
An Imprint of The Haworth Press, Inc.
New York • London • Oxford

Unbecoming Mothers
The Social Production
of Maternal Absence

HAWORTH Marriage and Family Therapy
Terry S. Trepper, PhD
Senior Editor

Unbecoming Mothers
The Social Production of Maternal Absence

Diana L. Gustafson, RN, MEd, PhD
Editor

The Haworth Clinical Practice Press™
An Imprint of The Haworth Press, Inc.
New York • London • Oxford

For more information on this book or to order, visit
http://www.haworthpress.com/store/product.asp?sku=5177

or call 1-800-HAWORTH (800-429-6784) in the United States
and Canada or (607) 722-5857 outside the United States and Canada

or contact orders@HaworthPress.com

Published by

The Haworth Clinical Practice Press™, an imprint of The Haworth Press, Inc., 10 Alice Street,
Binghamton, NY 13904-1580.

Identities and circumstances of individuals discussed in this book have been changed to protect
confidentiality.

Cover design by Lora Wiggins.

Library of Congress Cataloging-in-Publication Data

Unbecoming mothers : the social production of maternal absence / Diana L. Gustafson, editor
    p. cm.
  Includes bibliographical references and index.
  ISBN 0-7890-2452-7 (hard : alk. paper)
  ISBN 0-7890-2453-5 (soft : alk. paper)
  1. Absentee mothers. 2. Motherhood. I. Gustafson, Diana L.

HQ759.3.U63 2005
306.874'3—dc22

                              2004016529

Together and apart
Always in my heart
Amy (my BWBC) and Brad (my BWBB)

CONTENTS

ABOUT THE EDITOR

Diana L. Gustafson, RN, MEd, PhD, is Assistant Professor of Social Sciences and Health in the Faculty of Medicine, Division of Community Health at Memorial University of Newfoundland, Canada, where she teaches about health-related social justice issues. She has presented her research at numerous national and international conferences and published several articles on motherwork and other forms of paid and unpaid caring labor in peer-reviewed journals. She is the editor of *Care and Consequences: The Impact of Health Care Reform,* which has been on the required reading list of sociology, health studies, and women's studies curricula at several Canadian universities.

CONTRIBUTORS

Robert Adamoski chairs and teaches in the criminology department at Kwantlen University College in Surrey, Canada. His research focuses on the early welfare state and the child welfare policies in various historical eras. He is co-editor of *Contesting Canadian Citizenship: Historical Readings* (2003), which examines the citizenship construct in twentieth-century Canada.

Linda L. Anderson has a counseling practice that focuses primarily on issues of childhood abuse. Linda studied theater at Southern Illinois University and the University of Illinois. She is the senior administrative assistant in the Women's and Gender Studies Program at Yale University. Gardening, animals, children, and the sea call to her.

Susanna Calkins is a lecturer in history at Lake Forest College in Illinois. She received her PhD in European history from Purdue University. She is currently working on a book about the political activities of Quaker women in late seventeenth-century England.

Marilyn Callahan is a professor emeritus in the School of Social Work at the University of Victoria, Canada. She has published extensively on the impact of child welfare policies and practices on social workers, mothers, and youth. Currently, she is working on three related research projects: one focusing on grandmothers raising grandchildren, another examining the impact of risk assessment in child welfare, and a third on the representation of fathers in child welfare.

Lena Dominelli is a professor of social and community development in the department of social work studies at the University of Southampton, UK, and is also the past president of the International Association of Schools of Social Work. She has worked as a community worker, social worker, and probation officer. She has written extensively on antioppressive practices and the impact of globalization on human services. Her most recent book is titled *Feminist Social Work Theory and Practice.*

Patricia D. Farrar is a senior lecturer in the faculty of nursing, midwifery, and health at the University of Technology at Sydney, Australia, where she teaches women's health, primary health care, and research methods. She earned her PhD with a thesis titled "Relinquishment and abjection: A semanalysis of the meaning of losing a baby to adoption."

Barbara Field is a research associate with the Research Initiatives for Social Change Unit and a member of the Health Assessment and Resources for Children, a multidisciplinary child abuse and neglect assessment team serving Vancouver Island, Canada. She is a PhD candidate in the School of Social Work at the University of Victoria and has a special interest in the areas of women's health, substance abuse, parenting, and child welfare.

Lekkie Hopkins coordinates the women's studies program at Edith Cowan University in Perth, Western Australia. She is an archivist, oral historian, radio broadcaster, and teacher, and has been actively involved in the women's movement for more than three decades. Her work is feminist, poststructuralist, and cross-disciplinary. She is particularly interested in the storying of experience and is currently engaged in a longitudinal study of women peace activists in Western Australia.

Suzanne Jackson is a young, single, First Nations mother. The research project provided her with a great opportunity to address issues facing Aboriginal people every day while bringing them an opportunity to voice their experiences and concerns.

Audrey Lundquist is a hereditary chief of the Gitxsan Nation and a lawyer and researcher. She has a strong interest in Aboriginal rights, human rights, and social justice.

Gill Wright Miller is an associate professor of dance and women's studies at Denison University. She studied dance with Cunningham, Graham, Ailey, and Hawkins before accepting an academic appointment in Granville, Ohio, where she raised a family of four boys. Her choreography focuses on translating feminist theory to a physical experience. Most recently, Gill has published articles on postmodernism, body politics, healing, and public constructions of the pregnant body.

Deborah Rutman is an adjunct assistant professor with the school of social work and the senior research associate with the Research Initiatives for Social Change Unit at the University of Victoria, Canada. Her recent projects focus on substance use during pregnancy, adult living with fetal alcohol syndrome/disease, and young people's transitions from care.

Susan Strega is an assistant professor in the faculty of social work at the University of Manitoba, Canada. Susan's research interests include ethics, child protection, fathers in child welfare, and violence against women. She uses critical and feminist research methods such as discourse analysis. She has worked in many different social work settings, including child protection. Once upon a time, she was a "youth in care."

Si Transken is an assistant professor and chair of the graduate program in social work at the University of Northern British Columbia in Prince George, Canada. She is also a registered social worker who worked as a therapist for many years with women surviving abuse and violence. *Outlaw Social Work* is her most recent collection of prose and poetry. Her poems give voice to her experiences as a white bush trash girl/woman who knew various abuses and neglects, and to the perspectives and patterns she sees among her clients and students who have been hurt by a patriarchal, capitalist world.

Deborah Connolly Youngblood is a cultural anthropologist and author of *Homeless Mothers: Face to Face with Women and Poverty* (2000). She is currently a senior research associate at the Edgewood Center for Children and Families Institute for the Study of Community-Based Services in San Francisco, where she conducts research on child welfare.

Foreword

In any culture, traditional norms and patterns of behavior are established and authorized by the dominant social group. The expectation that mothers willingly remain the primary caretakers of their children at all costs is one such patriarchal norm. This assumption advantages fathers by removing the constraints and restrictions from their parental obligations, allowing them more flexibility, freedom, and control.

It requires courage and resilience to confront and resist the dominant status quo. Diana Gustafson has done both in this thought-provoking and timely documentation about mothers who choose to leave their children and their homes. Mothers remain central, it would seem, even when absent. By examining this phenomenon from multiple perspectives, this edited collection explores the complexities involved in making such controversial decisions, exposes the harsh realities faced by many women, and examines the unfortunate penalties and consequences imposed by a hegemonic culture. The personal stories and research studies Gustafson has compiled challenge readers to step into the invisible world of a diverse group of mothers and to consider their rights to full and fulfilling lives. In doing so, it dismantles and reconstructs realistic boundaries and workable patterns that could significantly change the regulation of women's lives as well as the evaluation of their acts of mothering. Each chapter emphasizes the need to recognize a wider range of social pressures, discriminations, and obstacles that challenge women attempting to raise children.

By creating secure spaces to talk freely and foregrounding experiences and voices of women struggling with depression or addiction, survivors of childhood abuse and poverty, lesbian mothers, single and teen mothers, or those called to serve God or fulfill career demands, these authors question the simplicity and inequity of the good/bad binary and expose the unspeakable grief, relentless guilt, and cover-up tactics that are central to a counterhegemonic discourse. The decision to become a mother is often shaped by societal expectations with far too little education and support for such a major life transition. It is no wonder that many women struggle with feelings of inadequacy, isolation, and regret. Motherhood and ambition are still largely seen as opposing forces.

As this book often points out, mothering is an identity and not a job. As such, it cannot be abandoned. Furthermore, a mother without her children does not mean that the children are without their mother. More often than not, mothers' actions to leave their children are informed by love and respect rather than personal pleasure. Even though mothers pursue options to benefit their children, they are branded as selfish, neglectful, unstable, and unsuitable role models. In fact, mothers are often forced to leave their children in order to access state welfare and support. Penalties for leaving children often include loss of custody and economic hardship.

The idealized maternal images of the "good" mother that we cull from religion, myth, fairy tales, and the media portray women as heterosexual, married, white, and middle class. They are devoted, loving, attentive, and self-sacrificing to their children. They are available, flexible, and asexual, with few personal needs to be nurtured or fulfilled. Their adult daughters often perpetuate this myth, keep silent about the realities, and passively accept extra responsibilities, interruptions, and economic burdens of child care. Gustafson has pulled free a few loose ends in this complicated knot and invites serious examination of the intolerance for diversity among women, narrow views of family structures, and the limited range of viable options available. Each chapter delivers the message that mothers need to honor their full personhood and respect their own needs before they can adequately attend to the needs of their children. The stories uncovered and the realities addressed in this book make it a significant contribution to the literature on motherhood and worthy of further consideration.

Sharon Abbey
Brock University
Canada

Acknowledgments

What an enriching experience it has been bringing together this collection! I wish to thank the contributors who shared my passion for this endeavor. To every person who shared her story in the process of developing these pages, I thank you for your courage and candor. My thanks to the publisher, editorial staff, and the production team for their interest in this project and attention to detail. I acknowledge with tremendous gratitude the support I received from Margrit Eichler, Debra Riggs, and Si Transken during the long hours of writing and editing this collection, and to Karen Martin *who knew me when.* Your friendship privileges me. To my family whose love is the gentle joy that sustains me, I share this book with you.

Chapter 1

Framing the Discussion

Diana L. Gustafson

Few mothers are more stigmatized than those living apart from their children. It is perhaps better to be considered an unfortunate woman unable to have children (Exley & Letherby, 2001; Miall, 1986; Pearce, 1999; Remennick, 2000) or a selfish woman who is voluntarily childfree (Gillespie, 1999; Letherby & Williams, 1999; Morrell, 1994; Park, 2002) than to be marginalized as a woman who would give up, surrender, or abandon her children (Dolan & Hoffman, 1998; Ebaugh, 1988; Edwards, 1989). In pronatalist societies, in which becoming a mother is naturalized and reified, unbecoming a mother—the process of coming to live apart from biological children—is variously regarded as unnatural, improper, even contemptible.

This book explores maternal absence within the social and historical context of parenting in Canada, the United States, Australia, and Britain. *Unbecoming mothers* is a term I use to characterize both the process and the quality of many women's experiences of living apart from their birth children on a long-term or permanent basis (Gustafson, 2001). "Unbecoming" captures the socially constructed process of moving from an authentic state of mother to a delegitimated category of bad mother or nonmother. Unbecoming is also a descriptor — one that implies that the process is inappropriate and unseemly. Moreover, unbecoming is a social descriptor that attaches to the woman who is regarded as unfit or unnatural because her behavior deviates from dominant Western social and moral expectations of the responsible (female) parent. One impetus for this book is to explore the impact of gendered, raced, and classed discourses of mothering on the process and quality of women's experiences of living apart from their children.

The statistical increase in maternal absence is another reason for studying the social construction of maternal absence. Today, more mothers than ever before are living apart from their children (Bianchi, 1995; Eichler, 1997; Kanazawa & Still, 2000). The idealized image of a married man and woman living together with dependent children does not correspond to the actual diversity in family structures in the countries studied here. Analyses of American, Australian, and Canadian census data, the American National Survey of Families and Households, and the American National Longitudinal Educational Study indicate that many changes have contributed to the diversification of family structures over the past century (Battle & Scott, 2000; Bianchi, 1995; Büskens, 2002; Stewart, 1999). Among these changes are (1) a decline in fertility rates, (2) increasing prevalence of nonmarital cohabitation or common-law relations including same-sex couples, (3) an increase in divorce rates, and (4) the increasing prevalence of reproductive biotechnology (Eichler, 1997).

Lone-parent families[1] are a more common family form, but they are not new.[2] Demographic studies dating back to the 1900s reveal that 8.5 percent of American children lived in lone-parent families (Eichler, 1997). Death, desertion, or migration of one parent, usually the father, were the most common reasons (Gordon & McLanahan, 1991, as cited in Eichler, 1997). During the 1960s and 1970s, the number of lone-parent families in Canada and the United States increased dramatically in tandem with divorce rates (Bianchi, 1995; Eichler, 1997). Because children typically resided with their mother after divorce, there were more mother-child than father-child families. Between 1970 and 1989, census data from Canada, France, the United States, and the United Kingdom indicate that births to single women significantly increased the number of mother-child families (Belle & McQuillan, 1994, as cited in Eichler, 1997). While births to never-married women created more mother-child families than did divorce, the number of father-child families in Australia and the United States rose faster than the number of mother-child families. By the 1990s, fathers accounted for 20 percent of American lone-parent families (Bianchi, 1995). In Australia, between 1989 and 1998, the absolute number of father-child families increased by 58 percent (Büskens, 2002). Given these facts, it is worthwhile to understand how women experience mothering away from their children in a world that values maternal presence.

The focus on maternal absence and unbecoming mothers—rather than on parental absence and unbecoming parents—highlights the powerful, persistent, and naturalized way of thinking about a woman's primary responsibility to care for her biological offspring. Parenting labor, like all forms of caring labor, is highly gendered. The naturalization of a mother's duty to care is strengthened by the visibility of a woman's reproductive capacity. Pregnancy and birthing are conspicuous biological events. The umbilical link between woman and fetus becomes the metaphor for mother-child bonding beyond the womb. This is exemplified in the way a mother's care work is described "in terms of ties or bonds signifying degrees of personal familiarity and obligation" (Thomas, 1993, p. 652).

Consider the concept of maternal bonding that connects women to infant and child care. No paternal equivalent in everyday language similarly connects men to the care of their children (Baines, Evans, & Neysmith, 1998). It is not uncommon to hear a father speak about babysitting his children, and this characterization tends to go unchallenged. Imagine if a mother were to speak of her child care activities in this same disconnected and nonfamilial way. The same language choice by women is at odds with the supposed naturalness of maternal labor and affiliation. Similarly, the woman who disrupts the maternal bond by living apart from her children threatens the deeply entrenched division of parenting labor and the idealized imaginings of the so-called traditional family.

Images of the traditional family are embedded in social, religious, and political institutions (Kaplan, 1992; Thurer, 1994). How women come to understand themselves as mothers is shaped by beliefs and practices reproduced in and through these institutional contexts. Women's experiences are shaped by their various social positionalities in relation to these institutions. Although burgeoning research illustrates the diversity of mothering experiences, we know little about the complexities of nonresidential mothering. This book contributes to this dialogue by exploring from feminist, historical, and postmodernist perspectives the process and quality of women's experiences of living apart from their children and how that experience is socially constructed as unbecoming.

Some of what we currently know about women's lived experiences comes from a handful of American studies sprinkled over the past two decades. Geoffrey Greif's longitudinal study of noncustodial[3] mothers was one of the first and most ambitious to date. In 1983, he surveyed 517 American noncustodial mothers with follow-up interviews with thirty-nine women in 1988. He reports that about half of these women are well-adjusted while half feel unhappy and guilty. These outcomes are linked to women's histories with custody, child support, alimony, and the legal system (Greif, 1986; 1987; 1997; Greif & Emad, 1989; Greif & Pabst, 1988). Helen Fuchs Ebaugh (1988) explores women's decisions to become noncustodial mothers as part of a larger study of role exit. She writes that women "who gave up custody" are stigmatized by strangers, acquaintances, friends, and family as " 'weirdos' who are 'totally irresponsible,' 'depraved and immoral,' or 'crazy'" (p. 159). Sweeping generalizations such as these make it difficult for women to feel good about themselves and their lives, regardless of the circumstances leading up to the family reorganization.

More recent studies bring a feminist perspective to the examination of women's narratives about maternal absence. In her prizewinning study of noncustodial mothers, Lynne Clumpus (1996) reports that custodial mothers—the most common form of lone-parent families—are characterized as fit while noncustodial mothers are regarded as unfit. This characterization sets up a false dichotomy that masks gender inequities in parenting. In another notable study of nonresidential mothers, Ginna Babcock (1997) examines women's strategies for maintaining a positive sense of self while coping with the social stigma of living apart from their children.

Feminist scholarship that constructs knowledge drawn from women's situated lives or "from the inside looking out"[4] offers one representation of reality (Auger & Tedford-Litle, 2002). Some policymakers, governments, social agencies, and family studies researchers advance another representation of reality that constructs maternal subjectivity out of the needs of children (Brandt, 1993). Absent mothers are linked to children's social withdrawal or "acting in" behavior (Fritsch & Burkhead, 1981) and negative changes in self-esteem and school success (Mulkey, Crain, & Harrington, 1992). Some studies suggest that adult children of absent mothers experience problems with attachment, self-esteem, and interpersonal trust (Carranza & Kilmann, 2000), and are more likely to report depression, suicidal behavior, and substance abuse (Juon & Ensminger,

1997). By extension, literature such as this constructs maternal absence through children's responses to separation from their mothers.

Considered uncritically, such evidence points to the negative consequences of maternal absence on children's short- and long-term social, cognitive, and personality development. Because a mother is held ultimately responsible for her children, her absence is implicated in the negative outcomes seen in her children. Explicitly or implicitly, such literature constructs the nonresidential mother as socially deviant, psychologically deficient, or a personal failure. Her pathology is linked to the severing of the mother-child bond and the disruption of the traditional family. I am not suggesting that negative outcomes reported in children in reorganized families are unimportant. However, I am questioning the explanatory power accorded individual rather than structural factors—those factors that assign blame to absent mothers as if the family operated in a social vacuum (Clumpus, 1996).

Individualist explanations for women's experiences are found in many disciplines. For example, Kathryn Morgan describes how individualism infuses the study of women's bodies and health. In particular, she argues that the medicalization of women's bodies and health practices regulates women's behavior and morality.

> In its most atomistic form, individualism is often carried out in principled, context-stripping ways so that differentiating systemic factors such as culture, race, historical location, class position, gender, sociocultural age, sexual identity, political position and disability status drop out of the picture altogether. (Morgan, 1998, pp. 100-101)

Similarly, the discourse of maternal obligation and responsibility is infused with individualistic explanations that locate parental responsibility within the body of the individual woman and away from the structural and systemic factors that shape women's gendered, raced, and classed experiences as parents. When individual blame is the pivot point for discussion, we learn little about how a mother's positionality structures opportunities for and obstacles to successful parenting (Taylor & Umansky, 1998).

The concept of mother blame and the representation of reality from which it emerges contribute, in part, to the process and the quality of many women's unbecoming experiences. Mother blame, similar to other conceptualizations of blame, emphasizes individual deficiencies (Arditti, 1995). This social construct is so pervasive that it penetrates family research by shaping the way that questions are asked, findings are interpreted, and policies are written. As Margrit Eichler (1991) points out, mother blame exemplifies the widespread gender bias in family research.

Mothers are blamed—whether present or absent—for children's experiences, concerns, and challenges (Caplan, 2000; Taylor & Umansky, 1998; Thurer, 1994). As noted earlier, mothers are blamed for negative child outcomes in lone-mother families. If attention to individual responsibility for parenting were applied equally to men and women, we might expect to see lone fathers scrutinized the same way that lone mothers are. There is not—nor should there be—a paternal equivalent for mother blame to explain why children are not flourishing under their fathers' care. The quantity and quality of attention given paternal presence[5,6] stands in stark contrast to the disproportionate scholarly attention to maternal absence in the reorganized family.

Amid this powerful body of literature that points the metaphorical finger of blame at individual mothers, some researchers offer another representation of reality from the outside looking in. A few noteworthy studies of parental nonresidence suggest that negative outcomes seen in children may be caused by circumstances that go beyond maternal or paternal absence as discreet, decontextualized factors. Parenting is an interrelational activity that plays out in a variety of social contexts. Race, class location, and other social differences, cultural values, expectations about family life, and access to support networks combine with individual characteristics of parents to create the environment in which children grow up (Ihinger-Tallman, 1995). The following examples support this assertion:

The levels of the absent parent's familial involvement (Spruijt & Iedema, 1998) and financial support (Smock & Manning, 1997), influence child well-being. Stigmatization directed at a nontraditional family by others, including medical professionals, negatively affects child well-being (Mueller & Yoder, 1999). Women's legal experiences with custody, alimony, and child support, and the quality of the relationship between parents postdivorce also have consequences for child well-being (Christensen, Dahl, & Rettig, 1990; Greif, 1997). Education and marital status also mediate the effect of maternal absence on adult socioeconomic attainment (Amato & Keith, 1991). Moreover, children who have sufficient and positive information about the circumstances leading up to the family reorganization manage better irrespective of their material circumstances or the reason for parental absence (Owusu-Bempah, 1995). These studies and others suggest that the family form as a discrete factor is less important than the context in which the family form operates. Lone-parent families operate within a social context that values an idealized image of the family. Every day, lone-parent families are challenged by the discourse of the idealized family that is embedded in government, legal, educational, and health institutions—a discourse that regards this family form as broken (Paterson, 2001). Every day, negative social messages play out in the lives of individuals and families, creating increased parenting challenges, a narrower range of options for support, and fewer opportunities for realizing positive outcomes.

This book attempts to bring together two representations of reality for a richer conversation about maternal absence. That is to say, the contributors examine some of the multiple factors that contribute to maternal absence and family reorganization from the outside looking in while offering a view of nonresident mothering from the inside looking out. The contributors share a set of five assumptions about maternal absence and the families that emerge from that absence.

First, parenting is highly gendered caring work. Women are expected to assume ultimate, if not sole, responsibility for parenting. Women more than men are marked as unbecoming when they live apart from their children in a long-term or permanent arrangement (Greif & Pabst, 1988). Although gender is a crucial category of analysis for making sense of mothering and motherwork, this discussion goes beyond an exclusive focus on institutionalized patriarchy or the axis of male/female, dominance/subordination to explain the unbecoming process.

There is a temptation to frame some maternal absence as women's resistance to the patriarchal institutions of marriage and family. This is not surprising. The increased attention to absent mothers coincides with an increased visibility of white, middle-class mothers as never-married lone parents (Eichler, 1997) and, of relevance here, white, middle-class women living away from their children (Büskens, 2002). Both groups of mothers disrupt the idealized imaginings of the good mother and the traditional family. An uncomplicated gender analysis—one that fantasizes a sisterhood forged by patriarchal oppression—is similar to early feminist theories that falsely assumed women were a homogeneous group. Critical analysis of maternal absence must take into account the multiplicity of women's lives and motherwork, and the complexities of negotiating the unbecoming process from various social positionalities.

The diversity among women is closely linked to a second assumption. Mothering is not a monolithic category. Just as all women do not share the same experience of *becoming* mothers, neither do all women share the same experience of *unbecoming* mothers. Whether living with or away from children, motherwork plays out in a wide range of social locations. Race, age, class location, sexuality, and other social differences shape women's relation to motherwork, their different access to material and human resources, and the range of options available for day-to-day support with caregiving responsibilities. Recognizing mothers' positionalities is key to rejecting the construction of a single, objective, neutral truth about mothering and motherwork. In its place emerge multiple, situated truths from a variety of particular locations and social engagements that shape individual and collective experiences of mothering and meaning making (Harris, 1993).

Some groups of women more than others are disadvantaged by social expectations for mothering, and these disadvantages shape the process and experiences of nonresident mothers. Some women who are differently abled or who have problems with physical or mental health need time for healing apart from their children. Some women leave their children in kinship care for purposes of study, work, adventure, and personal growth. Some women lose their legal rights to parent because of incarceration, allegations of neglect or abuse, or a history of substance abuse or addiction. In the following chapters, a critical exploration of local histories and situated practices reveals the complexities and contradictions of mothering hidden by these legal and social labels.

The contributors bring a third assumption to their writings. Maternal absence is not a recent phenomenon, although the modest scholarly attention to this issue over the past twenty years may give that appearance.[7] For decades, many groups of women living in Canada, Australia, Britain, and the United States have been separated from the daily lives of their children. Agnes Calliste's (1991) study of the racializing of women's caring work in the 1950s and 1960s illustrates how some black women left their children in kinship care in the Caribbean to care for other people's children in Canada. Women from the Philippines and countries in South Asia, Africa, and Latin America are also part of the organized trade of workers (Chia, 2000; Henry, Tator, Mattis, & Rees, 2000; Hondagneu-Sotelo & Avila, 1997).

Approximately 160 countries, including the United States, Britain, Australia, Canada, Saudi Arabia, and Japan, employ hundreds of thousands of overseas contract workers (OCWs) each year. Many OCWs are female heads of family who have few or no employment opportunities in their countries of origin. Attracted by wages two to four times what they could earn at home, women take jobs overseas so they can send a portion of their income home to support their families and create a better future for their children (Forman, 1993). Over time, the movement of OCWs has come to be facilitated by government and corporate interests at both ends of the trading relationship. OCWs constitute a cheap source of domestic labor in the host country while keeping the economy of the homeland afloat. Thus, the process and quality of unbecoming a mother are shaped by historical and regional forces.

These examples lead to a fourth assumption. Mothering experiences play out in local, national, and global contexts that are buffeted by political and economic forces. These forces simultaneously contribute to the process of unbecoming mothers and the restructuring of families. The local and global emphasis on cost containment and debt reduction means that the welfare state is undergoing dramatic change (Baines et al., 1998; Kitchen & Popham, 1998). These changes negatively impact support services for motherwork in Canada, Australia, Britain, and the United States. Talk about meritocracy and individualism becomes more prevalent in everyday discourse, as does the conservative mantra urging a return to traditional family values. The faulty assumption is that women who want to manage their motherwork will make choices that help them overcome life's obstacles. Although this is possible for some, many women already economically and socially disadvantaged spin continuously downward. During times of dramatic political and economic change, some women have even less support to meet the social imperative to mother well (Kitchen & Popham, 1998; McDougall, 1998).

The fifth assumption on which this book rests is the recognition of a persistent and widespread expectation in the Western world to achieve womanhood through motherhood and to strive toward the unrealistic ideal of the good mother. Some expectations to mother well are explicit and written into state laws governing marriage, parenting, and child custody. Policies and practices of child protection agencies show how institutions enforce rules that organize motherwork and a woman's relationship with her children. As Karen Swift points out, the facts presented as "self-evident" in public and professional discourses of child neglect contain both the "surface realities" and the "hidden realities" of how women's choices are regulated by institutional practices (Swift, 1998, p. 160). Thus, the everyday practices of child protection agencies serve the functional goals of the institution while enforcing the dominant images and discourses of the good mother held by the larger society in which the institution operates.

Some expectations to be a good mother are deeply embedded in social practices and reflected in everyday language and popular culture. Consider, as Ann Kaplan (1992) does, images of mothers and motherwork presented in the daily news, films, novels, television programming, and advertisements. Although these representations do not have the power of law, they shape the way women and men think, feel, and perform the physical, social, and emotional care work in families. From these sources, women and men learn what is and is not acceptable parenting behavior. Men and women have different relationships to these traditions that give meaning to their parenting practices. Moreover, the sanctions for failing to parent in the accepted fashion are also inequitably applied to men and women, as well as among groups of women. Nonresidential mothers challenge the complex and sometimes contradictory social expectations to perform the good mother role (Kaplan, 1992). Having declared the five assumptions underlying this text, I conclude with a discussion of the organization of the content.

Organization of This Book

This book is organized into three sections: Part I offers a critical analysis of maternal absence from the inside looking out by documenting women's lived experiences of how the dominant mothering discourses shape the unbecoming process. Too frequently, when a mother leaves, her story goes with her. As Di Brandt says, a woman must be the "subject of her own story rather than the unconscious vessel of others' needs" (1993, p. 163). She also says that women "need to claim subjectivity apart from the needs of others, particularly the needs of children" (p. 160). The five contributors to this section make a conscious effort to reinsert maternal subjectivity into the public discourse about maternal absence.

My own chapter opens this section with an expanded definition of unbecoming mothers. I assert that the concept of unbecoming mothers characterizes the process and quality of many women's experiences of living apart from their children. Drawing on family research and mothering literature, Chapter 2 shows how master discourses of becoming a mother, and the pervasive and decontextualized images of the good mother and the bad mother, contribute to the marginalization of women who do not fulfill their naturalized obligation to raise their birth children. I explore choice as a "problematic" that frames the social construction of motherwork and the limited range of options available to some mothers to parent well (Smith, 1987). In light of these limited options, the chapter highlights two coping strategies used by nonresident mothers that tend to reinscribe rather than challenge the good mother/bad mother binary.

Contemporary religious and medical discourses organize the experiences of adoption and relinquishment explored in Patricia D. Farrar's chapter. Drawing on the written narratives of eleven Australian women, Farrar documents mothers' difficult decisions to allow someone else to raise their children and the meanings they attached to that loss. Informed by the work of the postmodern feminist Julia Kristeva, these mothers' voices expose the unnameable and the unspeakable as their words provide the evidence for adoption as abjection: abject birthing, abject to her baby, abjection in/as reunion, and the emergence of themselves as abject mothers. These voices are powerful in their own right and deeply meaningful to Farrar personally as the circle of abjection is reflected in her own story of loss.

Psychotherapy is a familiar mechanism for healing and self-discovery. Linda Anderson's chapter is a "facilitated narrative" that foregrounds a conversation between the author, who is a psychotherapist, and Cynthia, who is a forty-four-year-old white, middle-class lesbian. Their conversation delves into Cynthia's identity as a mother and how those negative and painful feelings are intertwined with her sexual identity, childhood trauma, recovery from substance abuse, and recent diagnosis of multiple sclerosis. The analysis situates Cynthia's struggle for healing within the larger context of political and cultural realities that organize and limit some women's choices and their potential for an integration of their best emotional, spiritual, intellectual, and mothering selves.

Lekkie Hopkins' chapter is a multilayered exploration of pedagogy as a tool for healing and a re-storying of the self. Hopkins foregrounds a seminar presentation given by a student, Sandy Newby, about her process of coming to live apart from her children. As a feminist academic and teacher, Hopkins is fascinated by the ways we come to know and make spaces for diverse groups of women to speak and be heard. A goal in her women's studies classes is to challenge students' notions of personal identity as coherent, fixed, and predetermined. The students' task was to draw on their own experiences of being marginalized and to begin making connections between the self and the Other. One student's presentation about her unbecoming process had a profound influence on her listeners, creating a moment that both she and her teacher came to see as an epiphanous moment in the student's university life. The chapter presents the entwined understandings of a process of re-storying the self as an unbecoming mother and contributes to feminist understandings of the mind-body-spirit as epistemological sites and the complex fluidity of subjectivity and power.

Si Transken's use of poetry challenges the constraints of more traditional academic writing about motherwork. At the same time, she provokes our gendered and classed ways of constructing knowledge about mothers living apart from their children. Her poem links personal experience to the broader social context in which women live the contradictions of mothering. You will slip comfortably into her voice and find yourself responding to the authenticity and directness of her word. Then, she will unsettle you with the unadorned rawness of her story and the sharpness of her political commentary.

Part II looks at unbecoming mothers from the perspective of those on the outside looking in. The three chapters in this section critically examine some contemporary and historical perspectives on the process and the quality of many women's experiences of living away from their biological children. The chapters look at how the gendered division of parenting responsibility is constituted by and through religious doctrine, family law and child rescue legislation, institutional rules, and everyday practices. These analyses reveal the historical and contemporary marginalization of women as well as their resistance to Western discourses of mothering and motherwork.

Susanna Calkins offers a critical look at the spiritual and mothering selves of Quaker mothers from seventeenth-century England. Often journeying great distances across Europe, the Middle East, and North America, these women sought to fulfill their mission of becoming the handmaidens of God. In response to the scorn they faced for abandoning their children, many of them refashioned themselves as spiritual mothers who had been commanded by God to look after the needs of all Quakers, not just the needs of their own families. Through letters, testaments, and sermons, these mothers detailed their virtue and confirmed their value as prophets, teachers, and leaders. In extensive tracts, they outlined their expectations for motherhood and proposed ethical guidelines for raising children. Calkins argues that in the process of unbecoming mothers of their own offspring, Quaker women reclaimed legitimacy through new broader identities as spiritual mothers. In doing so, they simultaneously contributed to contemporary Western prescriptions for motherhood.

Robert Adamoski's chapter is a historical analysis of the experiences of lone mothers in Canada who came into contact with the Vancouver Children's Aid Society during the first three decades of the twentieth century. Correspondence and other data drawn from the case files of 154 families allow unique insight into the ways gender, class, and race shaped the options available to lone mothers seeking alternative forms of care for their children. A naturalized vision of appropriate motherhood presented barriers to mother-child families that did not characterize father-child families. Naturalized motherhood and the recourse to the language of human rights also infused the claims of these women. Ultimately, the struggles that surrounded child rescue cast important light on the nature of citizenship in the then-emerging Canadian welfare state as well as inform contemporary policy analysis.

Deborah Connolly Youngblood takes a contemporary look at the unbecoming process from the perspective of girls whose mothers are unable to meet "good mother" standards. Based on twenty-five open-ended qualitative interviews and anthropological fieldwork, this chapter explores the personal and social significance of absent mothers in the lives of African-American girls between eleven and twenty years of age. Girls who are being raised by relative caregivers are concerned that they are not being raised by their biological mothers, which affects their identity and self-esteem. The author argues that cultural ideologies that idealize biological motherhood are problematic for many constituents including young people in foster care. She discusses how reducing the emphasis on biological motherhood would better serve young people growing up in reorganized families.

Callahan, Rutman, Strega, and Dominelli also study the experiences of a group of women who grew up apart from their birth mothers. While in state care, some of these women became mothers. In these situations, the state serves as parents and grandparents to these young women and their children. Social workers are also expected to negotiate these difficulties, frequently amid conflicting and insufficient policies and procedures. The challenges are substantial, particularly since the behavior of young women as daughters can influence whether they are able to continue to mother their children. The authors offer a beginning theory that explicates the differences in unbecoming experiences among young women. Drawing on grounded theory, they assert that those who are able to look promising to their social workers are most likely to receive what help is available. The authors examine this process of looking promising and its effects of excluding the young women most in need of assistance. They include a critique of the various theories of "breaking the cycle" from social sciences and public policies that sustain this process.

Part III illustrates the richness and complexity of combining situated knowledges to the understanding of maternal absence at the individual and structural levels. What emerges is a textured picture of the social production of unbecoming mothers. All three chapters offer new ways of looking at the interconnectedness of women's beliefs about mothering and the family, their relationships to their children, and how they perform mothering practices apart from their children. Each chapter offer insights about how to challenge professional and public discourses about family structures that emerge from the unbecoming process.

Coming from another social location, Gill Wright Miller's chapter is the multilayered study of the unbecoming process as explored by mother and child with and through the creative arts. Miller tells the story of a woman who for many years worked full-time in two jobs: motherwork and college teaching. In order to regain her sense of self as an academic, this mother of four took what she describes as a two-year sabbatical from mothering. Upon her return, she involved her youngest son in the creation of a dance work that explores what it means to be what her son called "away from home." The work was performed publicly in many places. The process of creating and performing together was an act of healing for mother and child. The mother/choreographer claims the time away is actually healthy for both mother and child, allowing them to renegotiate their relationship. She asserts that the concept of mother needs to be reframed as addressing multidirectional parent-child consoling, counseling, and learning rather than unidirectional parent-for-the-child laundry, dishes, and cooking.

Rutman, Field, Jackson, Lundquist, and Callahan present a critical examination of how Canadian policy deals with the issue of substance use, pregnancy, and parenting. This chapter combines the perspective of Aboriginal and non-Aboriginal substance-using pregnant or parenting women and the practitioners who work most closely with them. From this investigation, the authors identify some possible solutions that are less polarizing and punitive toward women and may address the circumstances that set into motion the unbecoming process. Challenging the assumption that women are choosing between a life with substances or a life with their children, the authors detail the effect of existing policies on substance-using women. This includes women's separation or fear of separation from their children and their ideas about approaches that would make a positive difference in their lives.

Collectively, these works illustrate the dynamic relationship between how women think about mothering and the family, how they understand their relationship to their children, and how they perform mothering practices apart from their children. Acknowledging the spectrum of positionalities from which absent mothers emerge adds support for a broader and more flexible definition of family. Revisioning mothering and families is important to women who must confront powerful social images in their daily work to redefine themselves in relation to the children with whom they no longer live. Revisioning mothering and families is also of interest to policymakers and community agencies working to respond to the expressed needs of women and their reorganized families.

NOTES

1. Throughout the book, I use the terms lone-parent family, lone mother, and lone father, rather than single-parent family, single mother, and single father. The term single can also denote a person's marital status, but the term lone is inclusive of single, never-married parents as well as once-married parents, now single through separation, divorce, and widowhood (Eichler, 1997). The term lone removes the reference to marriage as the only way to create a parent-child dyad.

2. Demographic studies provide empirical evidence of lone-parent families in North America dating back to the 1900s. Susanna Calkins's chapter in this volume (Chapter 6) offers historical evidence that some seventeenth-century Quaker women left their children in kinship care when responding to a spiritual calling.

3. The terms noncustodial mother and custodial parent are avoided for two reasons. Although these are accepted legal terms and a part of the everyday discourse, the concept of custody constructs the relationship between parent and child as one based on ownership of property. The term is also a misnomer as it is not inclusive of the variety of situations involving maternal absence. When the term does appear in this volume, it is limited to either a legally defined context or the language of a primary source.

4. I am grateful to Jeanette Auger and Diane Tedford-Litle for their insightful writings about insider-outsider research and the social construction of aging. They argue convincingly that knowledge on aging advanced by experts such as educators, policymakers, and social planners tends to construct a reality from "the outside looking in." Auger and Tedford-Litle argue in favor of including knowledge advanced by those who live the aging experience to construct another reality from "the inside looking out." I use this insight to construct more inclusive knowledge about maternal absence from both vantage points.

5. At the same time that modest scholarly attention focused on absent mothers, there was a dramatic surge in cultural representations of fathers entering the domestic terrain. Ann Kaplan characterizes the 1980s as the "decade for fantasies of the Father as nurturer" (1992, p. 184).

6. Geoffrey Greif's (1987) longitudinal study of noncustodial mothers included a component that assessed the effect of mothers' involvement on fathers' levels of satisfaction. Another study by Battle and Scott (2000) compared the relative academic success of African-American males raised in single-mother versus single-father households and found that the impact of family structure disappears when socioeconomic status is held constant. Also of note is a special issue of the *Journal of Family Issues* (1999) devoted to comparing the experiences and coping strategies of lone fathers and lone mothers.

7. Modest scholarly attention to absent mothers began in 1980s and coincided with two events: (1) psychological studies of fathers adopting more nurturing roles in the family and (2) increased media attention to fathers' victories in custody suits and fathers' rights in abortion cases (Kaplan, 1992). These two events suggest a "cultural reaction" to the previous decade known for women's liberation and other civil rights movements (p. 184).

REFERENCES

Amato, P.R. & Keith, B. (1991). Separation from a parent during childhood and adult socioeconomic attainment. *Social Forces, 70*(1), 187-206.

Arditti, J.A. (1995). Noncustodial parents: Emergent issues of diversity and process. *Marriage and Family Review, 20*(1/2), 283-304.

Auger, J.A. & Tedford-Litle, D. (2002). *From the inside looking out: Competing ideas about growing old*. Halifax, NS: Fernwood.

Babcock, G.M. (1997). Stigma, identity dissonance, and the nonresidential mother. *Journal of Divorce and Remarriage, 28*(1/2), 139-156.

Baines, C.T., Evans, P.M., & Neysmith, S.M. (1998). Women's caring: Work expanding, state contracting. In C.T. Baines, P.M. Evans, & S.M. Neysmith (Eds.), *Women's caring: Feminist perspectives on social welfare* (2nd ed., pp. 3-22). Toronto, ON: Oxford University Press.

Battle, J. & Scott, B.M. (2000). Mother-only versus father-only households: Educational outcomes for African American males. *Journal of African American Men 5*(2), 93-116.

Bianchi, S.M. (1995). The changing demographic and socioeconomic characteristics of single parent families. *Marriage and Family Review, 20*(1/2), 71-97.

Brandt, D. (1993). *Wild mother dancing: Maternal narrative in Canadian literature*. Winnipeg: University of Manitoba Press.

Büskens, P. (2002). From perfect housewife to fishnet stockings and not quite back again: One mother's story of leaving home. *Journal of the Association for Research on Mothering, 4*(1), 33-45.

Calliste, A. (1991). Canada's immigration policy and domestics from the Caribbean: The second domestic scheme. In J. Vorst, et. al. (Eds.), *Race, class, gender: Bonds and barriers* (2nd ed., pp. 136-168). Toronto, ON: Society for Socialist Studies and Garamond Press.

Caplan, P.J. (2000). *The new don't blame mother: Mending the mother-daughter relationship*. New York: Routledge.

Carranza, L.V. & Kilmann, P.R. (2000). Links between perceived parent characteristics and attachment variables for young women from intact families. *Adolescence, 35*(138), 295-312.

Chia, A. (2000). Singapore's economic internationalization and its effects on work and family. *Journal of Social Issues in Southeast Asia, 15*(1), 123-138.

Christensen, D.H., Dahl, C.M., & Rettig, K.D. (1990). Noncustodial mothers and child support: Examining the larger context. *Family Relations, 39*(October), 388-394.

Clumpus, L. (1996). No-woman's land: The story of non-custodial mothers. The Feminism and Psychology Undergraduate Prize 1995 prizewinning entry. *Feminism and Psychology, 6*(2), 237-244.

Dolan, M.A. & Hoffman, C.D. (1998). The differential effects of marital and custodial status on perceptions of mothers and fathers. *Journal of Divorce and Remarriage, 29*(3/4), 55-64.

Ebaugh, H.R.F. (1988). *Becoming an ex: The process of role exit.* Chicago: University of Chicago Press.

Edwards, H. (1989). *How could you? Mothers without custody of their children.* Freedom, CA: Crossing Press.

Eichler, M. (1991). *Nonsexist research methods: A practical guide.* New York: Routledge.

Eichler, M. (1997). *Family shifts: Families, policies and gender equality.* Toronto, ON: Oxford University Press.

Exley, C. & Letherby, G. (2001). Managing a disrupted lifecourse: Issues of identity and emotion work. *Health, 5*(1), 112-132.

Forman, G. (1993). Women without their children: Immigrant women in the US. *Development, 4,* 51-55.

Fritsch, T.A. & Burkhead, J.D. (1981). Behavioral reactions of children to parental absence due to imprisonment. *Family Relations, 30*(1), 83-88.

Gillespie, R. (1999). Voluntary childlessness in the United Kingdom. *Reproductive Health Matters, 7*(13), 43-53.

Greif, G.L. (1986). Mothers without custody and child support. *Family Relations, 35*(January), 87-93.

Greif, G.L. (1987). Mothers without custody. *Social Work, 32*(1), 11-16.

Greif, G.L. (1997). Working with noncustodial mothers. *Families in Society: The Journal of Contemporary Human Services, 78*(January-February), 46-52.

Greif, G.L. & Emad, F. (1989). A longitudinal examination of mothers without custody: Implications for treatment. *The American Journal of Family Therapy, 17*(2), 155-163.

Greif, G.L. & Pabst, M.S. (1988). *Mothers without custody? "How could a mother do such a thing?"* Lexington, MA: Lexington Books.

Gustafson, D.L. (2001). Unbecoming behaviour: One woman's story of becoming a non-custodial mother. *Journal of the Association for Research on Mothering, 3*(1), 203-212.

Harris, C.I. (1993). Whiteness as property. *Harvard Law Review, 106*(8), 1707-1791.

Henry, F., Tator, C., Mattis, W., & Rees, T. (2000). *The colour of democracy: Racism in Canadian society* (2nd ed.). Toronto, ON: Harcourt Brace and Co.

Hondagneu-Sotelo, P. & Avila, E. (1997). "I'm here, but I'm there": The meanings of Latina transnational motherhood. *Zero to Three, 11*(5), 548-571.

Ihinger-Tallman, M. (1995). Quality of life and well-being of single parent families: Disparate voices or a long overdue chorus? *Marriage and Family Review, 20*(3/4), 513-532.

Juon, H.S. & Ensminger, M.E. (1997). Childhood, adolescent, and young adult predictors of suicidal behaviors: A prospective study of African Americans. *The Journal of Child Psychology and Psychiatry and Allied Disciplines, 38*(July), 553-563.

Kanazawa, S. & Still, M.C. (2000). Parental investment as a game of chicken. *Politics and Life Sciences, 19*(1), 17-26.

Kaplan, E.A. (Ed.). (1992). *Motherhood and representation: The mother in popular culture and melodrama*. London: Routledge.

Kitchen, B. & Popham, R. (1998). The attack on motherwork in Ontario. In L. Ricciutelli, J. Larkin, & E. O'Neill (Eds.), *Confronting the cuts: A sourcebook for women in Ontario* (pp. 45-56). Toronto, ON: Inanna Publications.

Letherby, G. & Williams, C. (1999). Non-motherhood: Ambivalent autobiographies. *Feminist Studies, 25*(3), 719-728.

McDougall, P. (1998). Confronting the cuts: One woman's story. In L. Ricciutelli, J. Larkin, & E. O'Neill (Eds.), *Confronting the cuts: A sourcebook for women in Ontario* (pp. 99-102). Toronto, ON: Inanna Publications.

Miall, C. (1986). The stigma of involuntary childlessness. *Social Problems, 33*(4), 268-282.

Morgan, K.P. (1998). Contested bodies, contested knowledges: Women, health, and the politics of medicalization. In S. Sherwin (Ed.), *The politics of women's health: Exploring agency and autonomy* (pp. 83-121). Philadelphia: Temple University Press.

Morrell, C. (1994). *Unwomanly conduct: The challenges of intentional childlessness*. New York: Routledge.

Mueller, K.A. & Yoder, J.D. (1999). Stigmatization of non-normative family size status. *Sex Roles, 41*(11/12), 901-919.

Mulkey, L.M., Crain, R.L., & Harrington, A.J.C. (1992). One-parent households and achievement: Economic and behavioral. *Sociology of Education, 65*(1), 48-65.

Owusu-Bempah, J. (1995). Information about the absent parent as a factor in the well-being of children of single-parent families. *International Social Work, 38*(3), 253-275.

Park, K. (2002). Stigma management among the voluntarily childless. *Sociological Perspectives, 45*(1), 21-45.

Paterson, W.A. (2001). *Unbroken homes: Single-parent mothers tell their stories*. Binghamton, NY: The Haworth Press.

Pearce, T.O. (1999). She will not be listened to in public: Perceptions among the Yoruba of infertility and childlessness in women. *Reproductive Health Matters, 7*(13), 69-79.

Remennick, L. (2000). Childless in the land of imperative motherhood: Stigma and coping among infertile Israeli women. *Sex Roles, 43*(11/12), 821-841.

Smith, D.E. (1987). *The everyday world as problematic: A feminist sociology*. Toronto, ON: University of Toronto Press.

Smock, P.J. & Manning, W.D. (1997). Nonresident parents' characteristics and child support. *Journal of Marriage and the Family, 59*(4), 798-808.

Spruijt, E. & Iedema, J. (1998). Well being of youngsters of divorce without contact with nonresident parents in the Netherlands. *Journal of Comparative Family Studies, 29*(3), 517-527.

Stewart, S.D. (1999). Nonresident mothers' and fathers' social contact with children. *Journal of Marriage and the Family, 61*(4), 894-907.

Swift, K. (1998). Contradictions in child welfare: Neglect and responsibility. In C.T. Baines, P.M. Evans, & S.M. Neysmith (Eds.), *Women's caring: Feminist perspectives on social welfare* (2nd ed., pp. 160-187). Toronto, ON: Oxford University Press.

Taylor, M.L. & Umansky, L. (Eds.). (1998). *"Bad" mothers: The politics of blame in twentieth-century America.* New York: New York University Press.

Thomas, C. (1993). De-constructing concepts of care. *Sociology, 27*(4), 649-669.

Thurer, S.L. (1994). *The myths of motherhood: How culture reinvents the good mother.* New York: Houghton-Mifflin.

PART I:
PERSPECTIVES FROM THE INSIDE LOOKING OUT

Chapter 2

The Social Construction
of Maternal Absence

Diana L. Gustafson

Unbecoming behavior was a term I used when describing one woman's transition from lone mother to nonresident mother—a transition that was regarded as "socially shameful and offensive to moral sensibilities" (Gustafson, 2001, p. 203). That case study documented the two-year period during which a lone mother decided to let first one, then both, of her children live for an extended period of time with their birth father. The process was reflexive and emotionally, physically, and financially painful for the white, middle-class woman who worked as a nursing professor in a large Canadian college. Ultimately, the process was shaped by her desire to find the best outcome for her children and herself. As she says, "I had to be a great big whole person in my own right before I could be a good mother to my children." Her difficult decision was compounded when she learned that her carefully considered reasons for arranging kinship care were not viewed as particularly relevant by some friends, members of her extended family, work associates, and the wider community. The fact of her absence from the day-to-day lives of her children was more important than her social circumstances in their negative assessment of her as a mother and a woman. Ironically, in performing what she regarded as the caring act of a good mother, this woman committed what others regarded as behavior unbecoming a mother.

This chapter contributes to our understanding of the social construction of maternal absence by exploring the process and quality of that woman's experience of living apart from her birth children. Revisiting this previously published (Gustafson, 2001) case study offers a view of maternal absence "from the inside looking out" (Auger &

Tedford-Litle, 2002) and complicates the dominant discourse of absent mothers as bad or unbecoming mothers.

Unbecoming aptly describes the process of moving from the naturalized, reified category of mother to the delegitimated category of nonmother. The process involves a physical, emotional, social, and, sometimes, legal shift in the nature and quality of a woman's relationship to her birth children. The concept of unbecoming also conveys the social stigma that attaches to a woman who is regarded as unfit because she is believed to be abdicating her maternal obligation and responsibility.

Drawing on contemporary mothering and antiracism research to frame my analysis of the case study, I argue four main points: First, the pervasive, decontextualized images of the good mother and bad mother contribute to the image of maternal absence as unbecoming mothers. Second, the image of unbecoming mothers is a negative template of the myth-laden imaginings of becoming mothers. Third, rigid dichotomizations of motherwork regulate the quality and experience of being a present and an absent mother. And fourth, some strategies for coping with the social marginalization of being an absent mother reinscribe rather than challenge the good mother/bad mother binary.

I begin with an overview of the master discourses about mothering, focusing specifically on the good mother/bad mother binary. This is followed by a brief review of the literature on the process of becoming a mother as a social imperative and an idealized but undervalued state of womanhood. This discussion explores how binaries operate as conceptually simplistic political tools organizing and regulating women's diverse experiences of motherwork. The case study of a white, educated, sometimes middle-class woman explores unbecoming a mother as process, work, descriptor, and choice. The chapter ends with a critique of two strategies used in coping with the challenges of living apart from biological children.

THE GOOD MOTHER/BAD MOTHER BINARY

"Master discourses" about mothering are those overarching social narratives that organize women's way of thinking about, interpreting, and performing motherwork (Kaplan, 1992, p. 8). Over the past decade or more, many feminists have begun skillfully deconstructing master discourses of mothering (Bassin, Honey, & Kaplan, 1994; DiQuinzio, 1999; Kaplan, 1992; Thurer, 1994). These master discourses about motherwork advance social expectations for women's connection with their children. One salient feature of this master discourse is the good mother/bad mother binary. Subtle and not-so-subtle images of the good mother and the bad mother serve as the benchmark for evaluating mothering performance. These polarized images are frequently at odds with the complex realities lived by lone mothers, poor mothers, and other women mothering from diverse social locations. Examining the good mother/bad mother binary as an analytical and political tool is helpful in understanding the social construction of maternal absence.[1]

A binary is a conceptual tool for dividing relative social phenomena thematically into polarized or oppositional categories. Oppositional categories set up fixed ways of talking about individuals and groups in terms of sameness and difference. Typically, binaries emphasize either/or, us/them, good/bad, superior/inferior dichotomizations reflecting the beliefs and values of the dominant social group. The features or characteristics of one category are advanced as the norm against which the other category is evaluated as deviant, aberrant, and Other. Polarized images of "us" or dominant and "them" or Other are reproduced in the media and other venues of popular culture and in institutional practices. Stereotypical images of dominant and subordinated groups come to stand in for an objective, neutral truth, or what Carol Harris calls "phantom objectivity" (1993, p. 1739). Although both groups produce images that reflect their beliefs and values, minoritized groups typically have less power and opportunity to disseminate images that may counter dominant views or contribute to a more integrated understanding of reality.

Frances Henry and colleagues refer to the overarching social narratives that dichotomize social groups into we/they categories as the "discourse of binary polarization" (Henry, Tator, Mattis, & Rees, 2000, p. 28). As a tool for interpreting the world, a binary simplifies the examination of relative beliefs and values by reducing the complexity of multiple factors into discrete, oppositional categories. A binary is, however, limited as an analytic tool precisely *because* it is reductionist. Explanations and experiences are oversimplified, and variations within groups as well as the overlap between groups are ignored. The pervasive and continuing use of a reductionist conceptual

tool serves a political purpose by minimizing the complexities of social phenomena, advancing master discourses, and regulating minoritized subjects.

Henry and colleagues' (2000) critique of the discourse of binary
polarization is helpful in exploring the construction of unbecoming
mothers. I begin with the arrangement of mothers into oppositional
categories of the good mother and the bad mother.

The Good Mother

The good mother is imagined as the normal and desired state for a
woman and female parent. Commonplace cultural images tend to
represent the white, middle-class subject as the embodiment of the
good mother. She is the woman who embraces the beliefs, appearance, and behavior consistent with white, middle-class, Judeo-Christian family values (Kaplan, 1992). The good mother acknowledges a
child's need for love, caring, and nurturance and puts that understanding into everyday practice. According to Shari Thurer, the concept of
mother love "has achieved the status of moral imperative" (1994, p. xvi).
The good mother is selfless and puts the needs of her child before her
own needs in all things. This selflessness can precede birth and even
conception.[2] The extralocal control of women's reproductivity associated with the medicalization of pregnancy means that the good
mother makes choices about nutrition, for example, giving selfless
priority to the fetus (Kaplan, 1992), the products of conception, and
even her ova.[3]

A child's needs are advanced as the good mother's raison d'être
because biological ties are presumed to bind together mother and
child emotionally, socially, and morally. To meet a child's endless demands for attention, the good mother in contemporary Western society is charged with the impossibility of rendering continuous, intensive care from birth to independence (Büskens, 2001). The good
mother is also fiercely protective of her child and is responsible for
ensuring a child's safety under every circumstance.[4] Maternal omni-
presence and self-sacrifice exact enormous costs on a woman's career
aspirations, social life, and personal needs, as Thompson's (1999) research on mothers of competitive junior tennis players reveals. However, accepting the inequitable burden of parenting labor and selfless
love is an expectation of the good mother.

Consider the ease with which we can call up stereotypical images of the good mother from films, soap operas, magazines, and other re/producers of popular culture. The good mother's omnipotence in valiantly overcoming all difficulties is the stuff of fiction and cinematic legend (Kaplan, 1992). Regularly, Western audiences are served books and films that remind women of the duty to be good mothers under all kinds of adverse situations. For example, in the film *Stepmom* (1998), a saintly woman dying of cancer hands over mothering responsibilities to her ex-husband's fiancée who, in turn, cheerfully gives up her glamourous job to raise the children. Even under such extraordinary circumstances, the birth mother and the stepmother-to-be must subordinate their own needs to the needs of the children. This image of privileged women who ultimately act in ways that are consistent with being a good mother confirms the power of this standard as one to which mothers should aspire. The idealized image of the good mother is reified or converted into an objective fact (Harris, 1993). From cinematic tales such as this one, women learn what is valued in our society and what is expected of the good mother. The persistent and pervasive cultural imagery converts the idealized version of the good mother into the desirable, achievable norm.

Only a handful of cinematic stories, such as *One True Thing* and *Anywhere But Here,* represent more honestly the layered, complicated, and imperfect realities of mothers' lives (Dennis, 1996). In these representations of motherwork, heroism is not a grand act. It is the ability to make it through another challenging day having erred along the way. Although these are more realistic images, they do not have the mass appeal of the fairy tale version of the good mother. Sentimental images of the nurturing mother continue to resurface, affirming the power and tenacity of the good mother construct.

The Bad Mother

In the discourse of binary polarization, the opposite of the good mother is the bad mother. Marked as different, undeserving, and Other, the bad mother is the woman who fails to reproduce white, middle-class, Judeo-Christian family values in appearance, the espousal of beliefs, and the performance of motherwork. Poor women, Aboriginal women, immigrant women, lesbians, and other minoritized women tend to be positioned as Other mothers on a short downward slide to the embodiment of the bad mother.

The bad mother is imagined to ignore, trivialize, or reject her child's need for love, caring, and nurturance both as an intellectual understanding and as a lived practice. She is regarded as unloving and uncaring. The stereotypical image of the bad mother that springs to mind is the woman who neglects, abuses, or fails to protect her child. A woman who is unwilling or unable to perform her motherly duties is thought to be motivated by selfishness, self-absorption, and self-indulgence—all individual defects. Finally and germane to this discussion, the bad mother is the absent mother—absent emotionally or absent physically from her children. Given these ways of thinking and talking about mothering, a woman who lives apart from her birth children would seem to be the epitome of the bad mother—an unnatural, aberrant women.

In this passage drawn from the case study, the polarization of the good mother/bad mother is evident in this woman's recollection of the day she told her work colleagues that her children were living with their birth father and his new wife.

> Colleagues who had not previously engaged me in discussions of a personal nature were intrigued by my decision. The questions were variously phrased but the implications were clear. Why weren't the children living with me? Had the courts awarded custody to the father? Had I abused them? Had I neglected them? Was I unfit for some other reason? Did I have a "problem" with alcohol? Did I have a history of drug abuse? When I denied these causes for a change in custody, their questions took on a different tone. If there were no grounds for removing the children from my care, then why weren't they still with me? My simple answer was that the children wanted to live with their dad. Children want to do lots of things, I was told, but that doesn't mean that they get to decide where they live! Clearly I was abdicating my motherly duty to raise my children. Or perhaps, came the insinuation, there was a more ugly explanation. Was I using my children's feelings as a cover for my own deep-seated desires to be childless and carefree? Was I putting my own needs before those of my children? What other reason could I have for downloading the care of my children to another

woman? In any case I was unfit to parent and the children were better off with their father. (Gustafson, 2001, pp. 207-208)

Over the years, Western audiences have been served memorable caricatures of the bad mother. Numerous fictionalized tales tell of failed mothers who are blamed (mistakenly, I would argue) for having too many children, too much responsibility, too few options, too little money, and too little social support. Mothers also fail through their physical or emotional absence as illustrated in fiction (MacDonald, 1980; Suarez, 1991) and children's literature (Warner, 1996). Fairy tales depend for their drama on the unfortunate events that befall children whose mothers are absent.

Although a mother's absence implies that her role is vital to a child's well-being, mothers are seldom important enough to be cast as the protagonist in movies and books. As Di Brandt observes, "mother as subject and character of her own story, has been repeatedly suppressed and edited out of the canon of Western literature" (1993, p. 157). Consequently, what we learn from popular representations of mothers and maternal absence tends to be from the perspective of those, particularly children, who are left behind rather than from the perspective of mothers who leave.

The good mother/bad mother binary compresses mothering into oppositional or polarized categories.[5] This binary falsely represents mothering experiences as static or unaffected by social and economic conditions. Ahistorical and rigid categorizations of the good mother and the bad mother hide the fluidity of maternal experiences over time and across diverse groups of mothers. Despite women's diverse positionalities, master discourses homogenize mothering into two apparently discrete and monolithic categories.

Although dichotomizing mothers into good (present and fit) and bad (absent and unfit) is neither accurate nor fair, this false binary functions to regulate mothering identities and encourage conformity. Focusing on the desirability of achieving membership in the good mother category obscures the often subtle, assimilationist processes through which these misrepresentations become part of cultural knowledge and practice. Although some evidence indicates that family research and popular culture offer alternative images, the idealized image of the good mother persists as the unrealistic goal when becoming a mother and when being labeled as an unbecoming mother. I turn now to an overview of the process of becoming a mother and how it serves as a template for a negative imagining of maternal absence or the unbecoming mother.

THE BINARY OF BECOMING/UNBECOMING MOTHERS

Becoming a Mother

Becoming a mother is the process of entering into a state of motherhood. Becoming a mother is considered a normal part of a woman's experience and identity formation. Given the blatant and more subtle social pressures to achieve womanhood through motherhood, it is little wonder that many girls and women accept, with or without reflection, the expectation to become mothers (Gustafson, 1998). Indeed, becoming a mother is a highly visible demonstration that a woman is assuming normal (female) adult responsibility for a legitimate, if not always socially valued, form of caring labor. That is to say, normal, respectable girls grow up, get married, and have children. Studies show that women who are childfree[6] face considerable pressure from family, friends, and strangers either to have children or to explain their decision not to (Lang, 1991; Morrell, 1994; Veevers, 1980). Di Brandt argues that becoming a mother is advanced as a "biological and/or patriarchally imposed necessity" rather than the "conscious, intentional option" that it might be (1993, p. 157). There are some notable exceptions to this social imperative.

Becoming a mother is regarded as a respectable thing to do *if* a woman fits the image of the good mother. If motherhood occurs within the parameters of a committed, heterosexual relationship, the woman is accorded a measure of respectability and the event is marked with baby showers, naming ceremonies, and other social and religious rituals.

By contrast—and this is the power of oppositional representations—becoming a mother is less well regarded by the wider society if a woman is not the embodiment of the white, middle-class subject (Kaplan, 1992). Historically, this was the case for many women who were unmarried or cohabiting (Eichler, 1997; Petrie, 1998). This continues to be the case for women who are differently abled or chronically ill (Blackford, 1998), poor, or worse yet, poor with other children (Hanson, Heims, & Julian, 1995; LaMastro, 2001; McFadden, 1994),[7] a teen (Hanson et al., 1995), a lesbian (Arnup, 1998), an immigrant, a refugee, or a member of another racialized minority (Brandt, 1993; Forman, 1993). Generally, these women face a range of reactions from benign disapproval to social isolation or, in the case of women who are incarcerated or have psychiatric disorders, the loss of their right to parent (Hanson et al., 1995; Martin, 1990; Thomas & Tori, 1999). The range and intensity of reactions vary over time, place, and diverse social collectives. Given this caveat about the women who fit the image of the good mother and are lauded for becoming a mother—and by contrast the women who are the embodiment of the bad mother and are discouraged from becoming mothers—a number of myths exist about becoming a mother.

Becoming a mother is a glorified, myth-laden process as Shari Thurer (1994) thoughtfully details. The discourse of becoming a mother includes stories of joy, wonderment, and idyllic mother-child bonding. Although these descriptors are true for many, becoming a mother can also provoke feelings of shock, fear, ambivalence, and confusion (Gustafson, 1998). Many women are unprepared, ill equipped, and overwhelmed by the unexpected responsibility of motherwork. Motherwork consumes so many aspects of everyday life that many women feel they lose more than their freedom. They lose a sense of an independent self. Living away from children relieves women of the day-to-day responsibilities for mothering as the following citation from the case study illustrates:

> As time went on, I settled into my home, my job and my new life. With this came access to a set of social privileges that were, until that time, unfamiliar to me. I began to enjoy the freedom of staying late at work when I pleased; accepting a last minute invitation to dinner; ignoring the laundry when it spilled over the basket; watching a television program without having to negotiate with anyone. (Gustafson, 2001, p. 210)

The personal losses that women accept as part of motherwork are revealed by the increased independence associated with maternal absence. Acknowledging the pleasure that comes with greater personal freedom can be offset by feelings of guilt when the guilty pleasure comes as a direct result of reducing the maternal obligation (Forman, 1993; Greif, 1987).

Mothering subsumes a woman's identity in a way that fathering does not do to men. Many women have, and many more hide, feelings of guilt when becoming a mother seems to be at odds with the romantic ideal. The process of becoming a mother and assuming the responsibilities of motherwork is rife with contradictions between the ideology and practice—between the imagined and the lived experience of mothering. The discourse of binary polarization allows little space for appearances or experiences that fall short of the ideal imaginings of becoming mothers. The ideal of becoming a mother is invoked in constructing a polarized opposite of the absent mother as the unbecoming mother.

Unbecoming a Mother

Unbecoming mothers is the concept I am using to characterize the process and the quality of some women's experiences of living apart from their birth children on a long-term or permanent basis. Unbecoming captures the process of moving from an authentic state of mother to a delegitimated category of bad mother or nonmother, from being an insider among mothers to an outsider. Unbecoming is also an apt descriptor of the process—one that implies that the transition from present mother to absent or nonresident mother is inappropriate and unseemly. The transition is regarded as a matter of individual choice in much the same way that becoming a mother is considered a matter of individual choice. This is not surprising given the discourse of individualism that pervades Western ways of thinking (Henry et al., 2000). Thus, unbecoming is a social descriptor that attaches to the women whose decision to live apart from their children deviates from dominant social and moral expectations of the responsible female parent.

The incidence of maternal absence is increasing and contributes to the growing diversity in family forms (Eichler, 1997). In Britain, 150,000 or about 15 percent of mothers were living away from their children in the early 1990s (Jackson, 1994). Toward the end of the twentieth century in the United States, the number of noncustodial[8] mothers was "close to three million" with "no sign that this trend will reverse itself" (Greif, 1997, p. 46). When mothers live apart from their children, it may be a permanent family reorganization or, as documented in the case study, a long-term arrangement lasting for years. The length of time women live apart from their children varies across time, geography, and social groups, and can depend on whether the process was initiated by the woman, the state, or jointly.

What circumstances precipitate the process of unbecoming a mother? The powerful and pervasive social expectations for women to be the primary caretaker of their birth children mean that the transition is not entered into precipitously by either the individual or the state. A common catalyst for maternal separation is the end of a marital or cohabitation relationship, when a child begins residing full-time with the birth father or another family member.[9] In these cases, the transition to nonmotherhood is marked by the courts and may involve protracted custody battles.

Custody awards are legal decisions that dictate parenting responsibilities for financial support and level of contact or child access. In Canada, these legal responsibilities are oriented toward the rights of the dependent child to receive financial and familial support from both parents (Eichler, 1997). However, records of legal decisions are not reliable indicators of how well a noncustodial parent fulfills his or her obligations to dependent children (Stewart, 1999a,b). Going to court to settle custody issues is a difficult milestone that affects parents, children, and their relationship with each other. Studies show that half of noncustodial mothers feel penalized by the courts (Greif, 1987; Greif & Emad, 1989). A passage from the case study describes the inequitable treatment one woman experienced:

> I had expected the custody settlement would be straight forward. Given our comparable annual incomes, I expected that my child support payments to him would be similar to those he had made to me. How naive of me to expect that I would be treated fairly! To avoid a protracted and expensive legal battle that would undoubtedly have impacted on my relationship with my children, I agreed to his demands to double the support payments. Each month I wrote a cheque for half my net income. And each month I was reminded that the courts mete out harsh punishments for mothers who "give away" their children. (Gustafson, 2001, p. 208)

Later she writes:

> When both children returned to live with me, the inequities in the way the courts deal with mothers and fathers were again vis-

ible. The child support payments required of my ex-husband were reduced to two-thirds of the amount I made as a noncustodial mother. (Gustafson, 2001, p. 212)

This experience is consistent with findings from Greif and Emad's (1989) follow-up interviews with noncustodial mothers. Half of those interviewed reported negative legal experiences or expressed bitterness toward the legal system.

Catalysts for the Unbecoming Process

Dissolution of a marriage or cohabiting relationship is one catalyst for the unbecoming process. Another is the birth of the child when a relative or the state assumes responsibility for the newborn.[10] Historically, arranging for the adoption of a newborn was held out as the best and only viable option for unmarried, white, working- and middle-class teens and women (Petrie, 1998). Today, adoption is still advanced as a reasonable alternative for women facing a variety of age-related, health-related, economic, social, and personal challenges. However, as Thomas and Tori (1999) point out in their study of women with serious psychiatric disorders, adoption carries with it far more serious emotional outcomes than choosing abortion.

Arranging for adoption, kinship, or foster care may come months or years after childbirth when a woman realizes that she is unable, unprepared, or ill equipped to raise her children. Other circumstances such as work,[11] education,[12] and physical or mental health of the mother or child[13] may also precipitate the transition to maternal nonresidence. Although systemic barriers to motherwork are not connected explicitly in everyday discourse to unbecoming a mother, poor or limited social supports for adequate food, housing, and child care make it difficult to mother, much less achieve the ideal of the good mother. It may be argued that women who agree to adoption, foster, or kinship care enter into the process voluntarily. As the following excerpt illustrates, the decision may be the best of many seriously flawed alternatives:

The custodial parent should be the one with the emotional and financial resources to raise the children. At the time of our separation it was I. Now things were different. Hours away from close friends and family, the pressures of building a career, a house, and a new family structure had taken their toll on me. My equilibrium was gone. Both children would benefit from living in a home with more emotional and financial resources. And so, with a mix of sadness and hope for my children's happiness, I said yes. (Gustafson, 2001, p. 207)

This passage also supports the assertion that women spend considerable time reflecting about their own lives, the well-being of their children, and what is best for all concerned before arranging for kinship care.

Sometimes, the shift in familial responsibility to state care is initiated by others who have the power to define or choose who constitutes the good mother. Rickie Solinger writes:

Government agencies, the courts and other entities have threatened, enforced, or terminated the motherhood status of certain women and girls, against their stated desires and without evidence of abuse because, for example, the woman in question was disabled, a political activist, too young, unmarried, comatose (judge denied abortion), divorced and had sex, too old, the wrong race, an atheist, a Native American, deaf, mentally ill, retarded, seeking an abortion, lesbian, reported to speak Spanish to her child, enrolled in full-time college, a drug user, poor. (1998, p. 383)

Even in these cases, the widely held perception is that women make poor choices that result in separation from their children. The mistaken assumption is that a responsible mother would not make decisions that might ultimately lead to court intervention. I return to this point when examining how the discourses of individual choice contribute to the negative social reactions experienced by some absent mothers.

Unbecoming As Process

First, I want to describe those reactions of family, friends, work colleagues, and the wider community. As mentioned previously, a woman's comfort with her status as an absent mother is determined, in part, by who initiated the process and by the quality of her legal experiences. The less control a woman has in shaping the process or a positive outcome for all involved, the less likely she is to feel positive about the transition, and about herself as a person and a mother (Greif, 1987; Greif & Emad, 1989).

The support of family and friends is another significant issue in shaping a woman's adjustment to living away from her children. Some factors are her relationship with the primary caregiver of the children, her relationship with her children, the age of the children, the length of separation, and the levels of family and community support. Many nonresident mothers are able to maintain a regular and meaningful connection with their children. Some mothers have their attempts to establish or maintain connection thwarted,[14] and some mothers have sporadic meetings or no contact with their children.[15] Some obstacles women face in maintaining a satisfactory relationship with their children and a sense of self as mother are evident in the case study.

> Negotiating access to my children was another regular reminder that I was a "bad" mother. Although my ex-husband had spent every other weekend with his children I found this an unbearably long time between visits. Unfortunately my requests to spend time with my children at least one day every weekend and one evening during the week were regarded as inconvenient and inappropriate. He said that children needed stability and consistency and that changing the schedule would be disruptive. I asked my ex-husband to consider the children's wishes. Children, I was told, weren't always in a position to decide what was best for them. The irony of these words was almost comical considering how my respect for the children's wishes had empowered their dad to deny them their decision-making. Nevertheless, I was restricted, with few exceptions, to seeing my children every other weekend. (Gustafson, 2001, p. 208)

Susan Stewart's (1999a) study of the relative frequencies of nonresident parents' involvement with their children shows that absent mothers are more involved in their children's lives than absent fathers. For example, absent mothers have more extended visitations and higher levels of telephone and letter contact than absent fathers (Stewart, 1999b). The higher level of maternal involvement may explain why young adults raised in lone-parent families enjoy similarly positive relationships with their mothers regardless of whether mothers were resident or nonresident during the child's growing up years (Aquilino, 1994). By comparison, relations between absent fathers and their children deteriorate significantly from childhood to adulthood (Aquilino, 1994; Kruk, 1993). Although the gendered division of familial obligation is an important factor in explaining the type and frequency of contact, further analysis of these data indicate that social location and circumstance of the absent parent are significant factors (Stewart, 1999a). For instance, women in more privileged positions have greater access to material and human resources that make regular and meaningful contact more possible.[16]

Unbecoming As Work

Maintaining a physical and emotional presence in a child's life requires a considerable investment of time, planning, and endurance, not to mention the instrumental work of mothering at a distance. Regardless of whether children are physically absent from all or part of mothers' day-to-day lives, children are seldom psychologically absent (Forman, 1993; Thomas & Tori, 1999). Many mothers who are connected by biology and disconnected by law or social circumstance carry with them the memory of their children. They maintain an emotional connection through rituals such as celebrating birthdays or keeping memorabilia that are reminiscent of those practiced by parents grieving loss by death (Abrams, 1999; Klass, Silverman, & . Nickman, 1997).

The responses of work colleagues and the wider community also shape a woman's adjustment to living apart from her children. Absent mothers tend to be viewed more negatively than absent fathers in terms of interpersonal adjustment, psychological deviance, morality, and professional competence (Dolan & Hoffman, 1998). Therefore, women who reveal their status as absent mothers may risk their job security and credibility. This may be particularly true in female-dominated professions such as teaching and nursing in which discourses of motherhood, femininity, and domesticity converge in institutional knowledge and practices that organize women's work and the workplace. Both teachers and nurses are described as having an obligation and duty to care (Achterberg, 1990; Noddings, 1994). In the United States and Canada, nursing education and professional practice standards merge the obligation and duty to care with instrumental or technical knowledge and skill. In Canadian educational law, for example, teachers are described as acting "in loco parentis" or as substitute parents in relation to the students they teach (Brown & Zuker, 1994).

The same discourses that structure mothers' work and identity also structure women's paid work and professional identity as nurses and teachers. When the nursing professor in the case study revealed her parenting status to her work colleagues, she simultaneously left herself vulnerable to questions about her professional willingness and capacity to care. This impacted her professional credibility and job security. I return to this point later.

Unbecoming As Descriptor

The responses of family, friends, co-workers, and the larger community influence a woman's adjustment to living away from her children. Many mothers also carry with them the memory of the conflict and confusion that characterized the process of separation and adjustment to a new family structure. Feelings of grief and loss—loss of what was or what might have been—are intensified by shame and social isolation at home, work, and in the everyday world. The living arrangement translates into and attaches itself as a descriptor to the woman, who is seen as lacking respect for herself and her children, as well as for her familial obligations. In her description of herself, this woman's words make powerfully clear the contribution of master discourses to the process of unbecoming a mother.

> My fragile physical appearance, my history of seeing a counsellor, my precarious financial state and my growing emotional distress over not being able to see my children began to shape my life in dynamic ways. To family, colleagues and the uninformed stranger, the reasons why my children lived with their father seemed increasingly obvious. I had become the image of the "bad" mother: self-absorbed, inadequate, out of control. When I looked in the mirror I could no longer see the "good" mother I believed myself to be. Gradually, my reasoned and reasonable explanations for not living with my own children seemed hollow even to my own ears. (Gustafson, 2001, p. 209)

Unbecoming As Choice

Master discourses convey a mother's obligation to care for and actively participate in the life of her child/ren, whereas a father implicitly has a choice rather than an obligation to care or participate in the life of his child/ren. A father—whether absent or present—who participates in his child's life tends to be valorized (Kaplan, 1992). A mother's expressions of grief and loss are delegitimated as a justly deserved penalty for abdicating her maternal responsibility. In the written narrative, the mother describes her feelings this way:

> Allowing the children to live with their dad was my "choice." No complaining was permitted for those who make bad decisions. My loss was self-induced. My pain was obscene. Noncustodial mothers were not to be embraced. They were to be rejected with contempt. These outcomes were justly deserved. The loss of that daily connection to my children was not recognized as legitimate. With little support, my grief intensified. I cried alone and ashamed. (Gustafson, 2001, p. 208)

These words show how the discourse of choice operates as a powerful element in the social construction of maternal absence as unbecoming. This woman implicitly argues that her choice cannot be isolated from the context in which she made that choice. At the same time that she is resisting the operation of choice, she acknowledges that it simultaneously shapes how others treat her and, in turn, how that makes her feel about herself and her decision. That is to say, the arduous day-to-day work of coming to terms with separation of mother from child is mediated and confounded by the socially inscribed responses of the legal system, family, and colleagues to the separation. Thus, the process of coming to live apart from biological children within a social context that valorizes the good and present mother ideal tends to construct the absent mother as the bad mother.

Comparing how maternal and paternal absence are characterized in everyday talk illustrates how choice operates as an important pivot in the good mother/bad mother dichotomy. Mothers who live apart from their children are said to *surrender* or *give up* their children. This way of talking frames the transition as an individual decision to abdicate primary responsibility for emotional care and support of her offspring. When a father leaves his children under comparable circumstances, the transition is not described using the same negative language.

However, a negative label is attached to some absent fathers. "Deadbeat dad" typically refers to the paternal subject who fails to provide financial support. The term does not extend more generally to the absent father's decision to live apart from his children, nor does it draw attention to any failure on the part of the paternal subject to provide familial or emotional support to children through regular, loving contact. Therefore, negative talk about parental absence highlights the gendered division of familial obligation as well as the differential attention accorded maternal and paternal choice as it affects children.

Feminists using the concept of choice balance the power of human agency that stresses individual ability to act and resist with the power of social and political structures to constrain social action. Blending the power of structure to constrain social action and the power of the individual to exercise control and make choices that embrace or resist master discourses is one way of making sense of the complexities associated with unbecoming a mother. The negative sanctions for failing to adhere to normative social standards for mothering may restrict the range of options available to some women. These choices are limited by institutional processes that embody and impart the dominant social discourses about women's social location in a hierarchically structured, pronatalist society. Although the concept of choice is contentious, one point seems clear: Regardless of how the process unfolds, the knowledge we have of maternal absence from the outside looking in may be at odds with a woman's definition of self or her understanding of the process from the inside looking out.

EXAMINING ACTS OF RESISTANCE

How do women cope with the multiple challenges of living apart from their children? Studies of childfree and childless women are useful in shedding some light on how absent mothers manage intrusions in their work and home lives. Childfree women, similarly to absent mothers, feel pressured to explain their circumstances (Park, 2002). Childfree women respond using a variety of coping strategies including selective concealment, medical disclaimers such as claiming biological deficiency, a process of "practiced deception," passing or identity substitution, and deviance avowal (Miall, 1986; Park,

2002). Most of these might be called defensive strategies. This section examines for the first time two defensive strategies used by the mother in the case study in her transition to nonresident mother: One can be labeled resistance through passing and the other resistance through selective denial. I discuss each of these strategies in turn.

Passing is an individual act of resistance directed at erasing an aspect of one's social identity or what Carol Harris describes as "voluntary surrender for gain" (1993, p. 1765). In her study of Blacks[17] passing as whites in a racialized society, Harris argues that passing is regarded as an act of necessity in the face of established social hierarchies that privilege some and exclude others on the basis of some real or imagined difference. Concealing social identity is an attempt to decrease psychological strain and avoid the delegitimation associated with the oppressed group. Assuming an alternative identity offers shelter from negatvie sanctions and the possibility of privilege and protection normally extended to members of the more legitimate group.

The nursing professor in the case study explains why she concealed her history as a nonresident mother. In doing so, she passed as a childfree woman.

> Relocating to a new town and job also allowed me to make new friends. Having learned a hard lesson, I presented myself differently. My experience taught me that acknowledging my children's need for a healthy, happy life with their dad could be twisted by critics into some sick kind of selfishness on my part. My agonizing decisions about the welfare of my kids could be translated by others into the facile act of "giving away my children" like they were unwanted property that I had cast off. I decided to draw clear separations between my personal and professional lives. (Gustafson, 2001, pp. 209-210)

This passage illustrates the negative reactions she faced at work for living apart from her birth children. Erasing her identity as an absent mother seemed a reasonable alternative to losing her professional credibility, her job security, economic stability, and emotional and physical well-being. When she took a new job, she made a conscious decision to present herself as a woman with no family, a woman whose life was her work. She writes:

> My emotional well-being and job security were too important to risk the probing questions and judgments of my new colleagues. Therefore, the desk in my new office was free of pictures of my children and other personal artifacts. These aspects of my life were no longer for public consumption. (Gustafson, 2001, p. 210)

She regarded passing as a childfree woman as an act of necessity that would decrease her stress and avoid the stigmatization and social isolation she had previously experienced.

Her decision to pass as childfree—a sad but selfish woman without the adult responsibility of parenting—seemed a more acceptable category of nonmother than her identity as absent mother—that despicable woman who gives away her children. Passing as a childfree woman or a nonmother is not without risks. Although concealing personal history preserves the self, it simultaneously denies the existence of children.

> By avoiding casual conversations at work about marriage, family and children, I protected myself from having to think about or talk about my children and my status as a non-custodial mother. (Gustafson, 2001, p. 210)

This act of resistance was motivated by her desire to protect her job and her health. By denying (through silence and performance) the existence of her children she escalated the shame she felt for living apart from them. In her own mind, she had reinforced the very image of the bad mother that she was trying to resist. Thus, the problem with this defensive strategy is the way it shapes the maternal subject and reinforces the stereotypical image of the selfish woman who would prioritize her own needs at the expense of her children.

The second act of resistance used by this woman can be labeled selective denial. By this I mean denying the image of the bad or aberrant mother by selectively calling up the image of the good mother. Throughout the narrative, this woman invokes images of the good mother when describing her transition from lone mother to absent mother. She tells about how she sought support from school officials, a physician, and a child psychologist. She describes repeated efforts to improve relations between the children and their father and his new wife. She details the emotional struggles leading to her decision to arrange for her children to live with their birth father.

How could I say yes? How could I say no?—Would a good mother not want what was best for her children? And it wasn't like she was going to live with a stranger. This was her father! What kind of hypocrite was I, the feminist, to say that simply because I am a woman that I make a better parent than a man, her father! Nothing made me intrinsically more suitable than him [sic] as a parent. We may not have been successful as husband and wife but I had no reason to think he was not a competent parent. (Gustafson, 2001, pp. 206-207)

This and previously cited passages reveal her resistance to the label of the bad mother. She describes her decision-making process, its consistency with principles of the good mother, and how that decision was understood by others as inconsistent with being a good mother. The implication is that she does not fit the image of the bad mother who lives apart from her children. Instead she distances herself from the Other by advancing herself as a woman whose thoughts, feelings, and actions are consistent with those of a good mother.

Resistance through selective denial intends to salvage the maternal subject by creating a new subcategory of the good but absent mother at the expense of reinscribing or Othering those "bad" absent mothers. Establishing new categories or definitions for good mothering by erasing and creating new boundaries around the old categories has the effect of reinforcing the binary polarization of the good mother/bad mother.

Furthermore, selective denial by creating a new, legitimate subcategory for mothering may be understood as a "race to innocence" (Fellows & Razack, as cited in Fumia, 1999, p. 90). By mobilizing and performing a particular white, middle-class subjectivity, some women are better able to represent themselves as the good absent mother while simultaneously distancing themselves from Other absent mothers who are framed as bad mothers because of their race/ethnicity, class location, sexuality, and so on. In her study of "mother-lesbians" Doreen Fumia describes motherhood as an institution "that regulates me into competing with other women on the margins of 'respectable' motherhood" (1999, p. 93). Although positive consequences accrue to those who are privileged by the new subcategory of good but absent mother, negative consequences accrue to those who continue to be positioned on the margins as the Other absent mother.

Resistance through selective denial is, in part, a challenge to mothering ideologies. Passing as a strategy for managing stress and social stigmatization tends to reinforce pronatalist norms. Both are defensive acts of resistance that acknowledge individual agency in the context of master discourses and structural penalties for women living away from their children. Both strategies are reactions to the stigmatized identity of absent mothers. However, both strategies are flawed as they reinscribe, in different ways, unbecoming as process, work, descriptor, and choice.

These defensive strategies do not challenge the assumptions underpinning good mother/bad mother categories. Neither response challenges the good mother/bad mother binary that regulates the gendered division of family work and parenting labor. Neither strategy reasserts motherwork as an impossibility for some women (DiQuinzio, 1999). Neither asserts a woman's right to live apart from her children. Neither strategy advances a woman's right to self-fulfillment and expression as separate and distinct from her motherwork. Nor does either strategy value the differently organized family structures that emerge when mothers live away from their children.

Proactive strategies such as those identified in Kristen Park's (2002) study of stigma management among childfree women may offer some possibilities for challenging dominant discourses of unbecoming mothers. Techniques such as preventive disclosure, condemning the condemner, and asserting a right to fulfillment challenge conventional ideologies about women and motherwork and redefine discreditable identities. If integrated into institutional and individual practices, these strategies may help to redefine maternal absence as a more acceptable social option in a reorganized family.

CONCLUDING THOUGHTS

The increasing incidence of maternal absence is part of the overall shift in family form (Eichler, 1997; Hanson et al., 1995). Over the past century in North America, Europe, and Australia, blended and lone-parent families have replaced the nuclear family as the most common family structures. Although many religious and other conservative institutions continue to regard the two-parent family as the ideal, if not the norm, some other social and legal institutions are redefining what it means to be a family.

Nonresident parenting situations are not generally regarded as a family form. Perhaps this is because absent fathers who make up the greatest proportion of nonresident parents are much less likely than mothers to maintain a familial relationship with their children. However, some nonresident mothers may constitute a family form because of the high levels of familial connection and motherwork. Thus, what constitutes the contemporary family may have more to do with the social interactional dynamics between individuals than with family form or structure (Arditti, 1995; Marotz-Baden, Adams, Beuche, Munro, & Munro, 1979).

Revisiting the case study of a woman living apart from her children illustrates that maternal absence or unbecoming a mother stands in conceptual opposition to the discourse of becoming a mother. Moreover, the narrative highlights the oppositional nature of the good mother/bad mother binary from which the stigmatization of absent mothers emerges. This white, well-educated, sometimes middle-class nursing professor uses two flawed coping strategies in responding to the social marginalization of being an absent mother. These acts of resistance—passing and selective denial—implicitly draw their power from a privileging of white, maternal subjectivity and a distancing of the self from other categories of so-called bad mothers. Unfortunately, neither strategy asserts a woman's right to live apart from her children or values a differently organized family structure. Instead, these strategies buttress the hierarchical ranking of mothering along race and class lines. This finding is a cautionary note to theorists who may be tempted to create new categories of the good absent mother that simultaneously reinscribe master discourses of the bad Other mother and the discourse of binary polarization.

NOTES

1. Ann Kaplan (1992) argues that popular representations of the good mother as Angel and the bad mother as Witch reflect and inform discourses of being and becoming a mother.

2. This is not a new prescription. As Susanna Calkins points out in her chapter, evidence dating to the Early Modern era shows that women were expected to protect their children before and after birth.

3. John Callis cites research done by a team of scientists from Canada, Australia, and New Zealand studying preterm births in sheep to support his assertion that women should eat nutritiously out of concern for their potential role as birthing

agents (Wong, 2003). Challis is quoted as saying, "Women need to think about proper diet and food intake before they even know they're pregnant because proper nutrition after pregnancy may not compensate for the lack of it beforehand. Even a modest restriction around the time of conception could have far-reaching consequences." The original study on sheep found that maternal nutrition at the time of conception was associated with long-term adverse health effects in offspring.

4. The significance of mother as protector was reinforced in a Canadian court in 1984 when a nonoffending mother was convicted of failing to protect her child from abuse committed by the child's father (Eichler, 1997). The courts held that because a mother is usually responsible for a child that the mother "should have known" (p. 221) that the child was abused. Since that time, the courts and child protection agencies focus on the mother and her role as protector rather than on the father and his role as perpetrator (Krane, 1994, as cited in Eichler, 1997).

5. The image of "good-enough mother," a concept coined by D.W. Winnicott in the mid-twentieth century, would seem to challenge the idealization of motherwork and the good mother/bad mother binary. However, some consider Winnicott to be "an ally in the project of valorizing maternal practice" (First, 1994, p. 147).

6. There is lively debate in the feminist mothering literature about how to name women who choose not to have children. Labels such as childless and childfree exemplify the centrality of the child in the construction of adult, female identity.

7. Recently, a bumper sticker was spotted in Reno, Nevada, that said, "If you can't feed them, don't breed them" (Betty Glass, personal communication, April 10, 2003). The underlying assumption here is that those who are poor have less right to have children. The implication is that the poor who do have children are a drain on the wider society.

8. In this chapter, I restrict my use of the terms custody, custodial parent, noncustodial mother, and so on to a legally defined context or when quoting a primary source. My understanding of maternal absence includes but is not limited to mothers living apart from their birth children as a result of a legal change in custody.

9. Lekkie Hopkins in this volume discusses living apart from her children following the dissolution of her marriage.

10. Patricia Farrer in this volume discusses adoption and unbecoming a mother in Australia in the 1950s.

11. Suzanne Calkins in this volume examines Quaker mothers in the 1700s who leave their own children to become spiritual mothers of their communities.

12. Gill Wright Miller in this volume explores the decision to live apart from her children while she pursues her education in another state.

13. Linda Anderson explores the story of a mother whose physical and mental health are major factors in her decision to live apart from her children.

14. Patricia Farrar in this volume discusses the problems of trying to establish and maintain contact with adult children.

15. Deborah Connolly Youngblood in this volume describes the family structure when mothers visit infrequently or sporadically.

16. The importance of social positionality is evident when comparing the unbecoming story of the mother who is a white, middle-class university professor (see Wright Miller in this volume) with the unbecoming stories of a lesbian mother (see Anderson in this volume) and a First Nations mother (see Callahan et al. in this volume).

17. Following the precedent set by Anderson and Collins (1992), I capitalize Blacks and not whites for political reasons. Black signifies the construction of color as a category of difference and flags the historical differences between the Black and white experiences.

REFERENCES

Abrams, N. (1999). *The other mother: A lesbian's fight for her daughter.* Madison: University of Wisconsin Press.

Achterberg, J. (1990). *Woman as healer.* Boston: Shambhala.

Andersen, M.L., & Collins, P.H. (1992). Preface. In M.L. Andersen & P.H. Collins (Eds.), *Race, class, and gender: An anthology* (pp. xii-xvi). Belmont, CA: Wadsworth Publishing.

Aquilino, W.S. (1994). Impact of childhood family disruption on young adults' relationships with parents. *Journal of Marriage and the Family, 56,* 295-313.

Arditti, J.A. (1995). Noncustodial parents: Emergent issues of diversity and process. *Marriage and Family Review, 20*(1/2), 283-304.

Arnup, K. (1998). "Does the word lesbian mean anything to you?" Lesbians raising daughters. In S. Abbey & A. O'Reilly (Eds.), *Redefining motherhood: Changing identities and patterns* (pp. 59-68). Toronto, ON: Second Story Press.

Auger, J.A. & Tedford-Litle, D. (2002). *From the inside looking out: Competing ideas about growing old.* Halifax, NS: Fernwood.

Bassin, D., Honey, M., & Kaplan, M.M. (Eds.). (1994). *Representations of motherhood.* New Haven, CT: Yale University Press.

Blackford, K.A. (1998). Mother to daughter: The shaping of a girl's values in the context of a parent with a chronic illness. In S. Abbey & A. O'Reilly (Eds.), *Redefining motherhood: Changing identities and patterns* (pp. 145-158). Toronto, ON: Second Story Press.

Brandt, D. (1993). *Wild mother dancing: Maternal narrative in Canadian literature.* Winnipeg, MN: University of Manitoba Press.

Brown, A. and Zuker, M. (1994). *Education law.* Toronto, ON: Carswell Thomson Professional Publishing.

Büskens, P. (2001). The impossibility of "natural parenting" for modern mothers: On social structure and the formation of habit. *Journal of the Association for Research on Mothering, 3*(1), 75-86.

Dennis, W. (1996, November 6). Mommy truest. *The Weekend Post,* pp. 1-3.

DiQuinzio, P. (1999). *The impossibility of motherhood: Feminism, individualism and the problem of mothering.* New York: Routledge.

Dolan, M.A. and Hoffman, C.D. (1998). The differential effects of marital and custodial status on perceptions of mothers and fathers. *Journal of Divorce and Remarriage, 29*(3/4), 55-64.

Eichler, M. (1997). *Family shifts: Families, policies and gender equality.* Toronto, ON: Oxford University Press.

First, E. (1994). Mothering, hate and Winnicott. In D. Bassin, M. Honey, & M.M. Kaplan (Eds.), *Representations of motherhood* (pp. 147-161). New Haven, CT: Yale University Press.

Forman, G. (1993). Women without their children: Immigrant women in the US. *Development, 4,* 51-55.

Fumia, D. (1999). Marginalized motherhood and the mother-lesbian subject. *Journal of the Association for Research on Mothering, 1*(1), 86-95.

Greif, G.L. (1987). Mothers without custody. *Social Work, 32*(1), 11-16.

Greif, G.L. (1997). Working with noncustodial mothers. *Families in Society: The Journal of Contemporary Human Services, 78*(January-February), 46-52.

Greif, G.L. & Emad, F. (1989). A longitudinal examination of mothers without custody: Implications for treatment. *The American Journal of Family Therapy, 17*(2), 155-163.

Gustafson, D.L. (1998). Learning to wear mother clothes to cover woman dreams. *Canadian Woman Studies Journal, 18*(2/3), 105-108.

Gustafson, D.L. (2001). Unbecoming behaviour: One woman's story of becoming a non-custodial mother. *Journal of the Association for Research on Mothering, 3*(1), 203-212.

Hanson, S.M.H., Heims, M.L., & Julian, D.J. (1995). Single parent families: Present and future perspectives. *Marriage and Family Review, 20*(1/2), 1-26.

Harris, C.I. (1993). Whiteness as property. *Harvard Law Review, 106*(8), 1707-1791.

Henry, F., Tator, C., Mattis, W., & Rees, T. (2000). *The colour of democracy: Racism in Canadian society* (2nd ed.). Toronto, ON: Harcourt Brace and Co.

Jackson, R. (1994). *Mothers who leave: Behind the myth of women without their children.* London: Pandora.

Kaplan, E.A. (Ed.). (1992). *Motherhood and representation: The mother in popular culture and melodrama.* London: Routledge.

Klass, D., Silverman, P.R., & Nickman, S.L. (Eds.). (1997). *Continuing bonds: New understandings of grief.* Washington, DC: Taylor and Francis.

Kruk, E. (1993). *Divorce and disengagement: Patterns of fatherhood within and beyond marriage.* Halifax, NS: Fernwood Books.

LaMastro, V. (2001). Childless by choice? Attributions and attitudes concerning family size. *Social Behavior and Personality, 29*(3), 231-243.

Lang, S. (1991). *Women without children: The reasons, the rewards, the regrets.* New York: Pharos Books.

MacDonald, S.P. (1980). Jane Austen and the tradition of the absent mother. In C.N. Davidson and E.M. Broner (Eds.), *The lost tradition: Mothers and daughters in literature* (pp. 58-69). New York: Frederick Ungar.

Mark, L. (Producer) & Wang, P. (Director). (1999). *Anywhere But Here* [Film]. (Available from Twentieth Century Fox, Twentieth Century House, 31-32 Soho Square, London W1V 3AP).

Marotz-Baden, R., Adams, G.R., Beuche, N., Munro, B., & Munro, G. (1979). Family form or family process? Reconsidering the deficit family model approach. *The Family Coordinator, 28,* 5-14.

Martin, M. (1990). Connected mothers: A follow-up study of incarcerated women with their children. *Women and Criminal Justice, 8*(4), 1-23.

McFadden, P. (1994). Motherhood as a choice. *Southern Africa Political and Economic Monthly, 7*(9), 40-41.

Miall, C. (1986). The stigma of involuntary childlessness. *Social Problems, 33*(4), 268-282.

Morrell, C. (1994). *Unwomanly conduct: The challenges of intentional childlessness.* New York: Routledge.

Noddings, N. (1994). An ethic of care and its implications for instructional arrangements. In L. Stone (Ed.), *The education feminism reader* (pp. 171-183). New York: Routledge.

Park, K. (2002). Stigma management among the voluntarily childless. *Sociological Perspectives, 45*(1), 21-45.

Petrie, A. (1998). *Gone to an aunt's: Remembering Canada's homes for unwed mothers.* Toronto, ON: McClelland and Stewart.

Solinger, R. (1998). Poisonous choice. In M.L. Taylor & L. Umansky (Eds.), *"Bad" mothers: The politics of blame in twentieth-century America* (pp. 381-402). New York: New York University Press.

Stewart, S.D. (1999a). Disneyland dads, Disneyland moms? How nonresident parents spend time with absent children. *Journal of Family Issues, 20*(4), 539-556.

Stewart, S.D. (1999b). Nonresident mothers' and fathers' social contact with children. *Journal of Marriage and the Family, 61*(4), 894-907.

Suarez, I.C. (1991). Absent mother(land)s: Joan Riley's fiction. In S. Nasta (Ed.), *Motherlands: Black women's writing from Africa, the Caribbean and South Asia* (pp. 290-309). London: The Women's Press.

Thomas, T. & Tori, C.D. (1999). Sequelae of abortion and relinquishment of child custody among women with major psychiatric disorders. *Psychological Reports, 84*(3), 773-790.

Thompson, S.M. (1999). *Mother's taxi: Sport and women's labor.* Albany, NY: SUNY Press.

Thurer, S.L. (1994). *The myths of motherhood: How culture reinvents the good mother.* New York: Houghton-Mifflin.

Ufland, H.J. & J. Beaton (Producers), & Franklin, C. (Director). (1998). *One True Thing* [Film]. (Available from Universal Pictures, 100 Universal City Plaza 1440/15, Universal City, CA 91608).

Veevers, J. (1980). *Childless by choice.* Toronto, ON: Butterworth and Co. Ltd.

Warner, M. (1996). The absent mother: Women against women in old wives' tales. In S.A. Egoff (Ed.), *Only connect: Readings on children's literature* (3rd ed.) (pp. 278-287). Toronto, ON: Oxford University Press.

Wong, J. (2003). Premature birth linked to lack of nutrition before pregnancy. News@UofT. Available at <http://www.newsandevents.utoronto.ca/bin4/030424a.asp>.

Chapter 3

Abject Mothers:
Women Separated from Their Babies
Lost to Adoption

Patricia D. Farrar

The number of women in Western societies in the twentieth century who have lost their babies to adoption is inestimable. In Australia and New Zealand the figure is in the vicinity of 200,000 (Harkness, 1991; Inglis, 1984). This number more than doubles when
statistics from the United Kingdom are added.[1] According to the U.S.
census, there were 1.4 million domestic and 200,000 international
adoptions in 2000 (Carangelo, 2004). It should be noted that these
data represent only those babies taken for adoption during one or two
decades, notwithstanding that this era represented the peak period for
adoptions. Moreover, there is little acknowledgement in the English
literature about European women whose babies were taken for adoption during the twentieth century (Farrar, 1997). Until recently, significant scholarly attention also had not been paid to the experience of
adoption and relinquishment from the perspective of mothers living
apart from their children.[2] Hence, the magnitude and meaning of this
issue is largely unknown.

This chapter examines the experiences of eleven mothers (including myself) who lost their babies to adoption and the meanings they
attached to that loss. Women contacted me voluntarily to share their
stories, some through an Internet adoption support group and others
after they heard about my research in the media. I asked them to write
their stories as a "stream of consciousness," recalling the events surrounding the loss of their babies to adoption. Their personal experiences are presented here in the words drawn from their written narratives. Their voices expose the unnameable and the unspeakable as

51

their words provide the evidence for adoption as abjection: abject birthing, abject to her baby, abjection in/as reunion, and the emergence of themselves as abject mothers. These voices are powerful in their own right and deeply meaningful to me personally as the circle of abjection is reflected in my own story of loss. Before I outline the features of Julia Kristeva's work that inform my analysis, I offer an overview of the literature on adoption and relinquishment.

ADOPTION AND RELINQUISHMENT

For almost sixty years the literature on adoption and relinquishment has drawn conclusions about women whose babies were taken for adoption (Farrar, 2000). In medical discourse the relinquishing mother was constructed as "mad." The reasons for her sexuality and extra-nuptial pregnancy were attributed to her defective personality and unresolved Oedipal conflict. Rarely was her mental state considered to be due to the physical, emotional, and financial stresses of her pregnancy. Problems associated with her mental health were presumed to reside entirely within her, with no contribution from or influence of social factors. When she was assessed in the postnatal period, her mental and emotional fragility were again attributed to intrinsic qualities: that the loss of her child to adoption may have been responsible for her mental state was not considered by theorists for many years. Any decision to keep her baby was regarded as pathological. To surrender her baby for adoption was healthy. Her pregnancy was considered a minor mental aberration that could be resolved by the removal of her baby for adoption.

Unmarried mothers were exhorted frequently that surrendering their babies was in the "best interests of the child" (Derdeyn & Wadlington, 1977), a phrase that has been enshrined in adoption and child protection legislation (Goldstein, Freud, & Solnit, 1973). The prime reason for the adoption mandate was not only that the child would have two parents but also that she or he would be as "if born to them" in a reconstructed nuclear family. Through the appropriation of their reproductive economy for adoption, unmarried mothers were assured that they were acting responsibly.

The unmarried mother moved from the construction by medical discourses as "mad" to a socially discursive space of deviance as the "bad girl." The so-called bad girl could be rehabilitated in a maternity home and then morally reinstated in society without her baby as evidence of her misdemeanor (Rains, 1970). A profile of the mother who surrendered her baby was constructed with two purposes: (1) to justify the rehabilitative practice of taking her baby and (2) in a buyer's market, to procure the best available babies for adoption. The mold was cast; all that remained was to fill it with the abundance of available clay so that the desirable mother could be reproduced and her equally desirable baby procured. The inverse model, the mother who kept her baby, was so negatively contrived that her baby was considered unwanted and unsuitable for adoption anyway, analogous to those whom the Canadian writer Margaret Atwood, in her novel *The Handmaid's Tale,* has called "the Unbabies" (1987, p.123).

During the 1960s and early 1970s in the United States, Gill noted an increase in the number of extra-nuptial pregnancies to women in upper socioeconomic groups (1977). Despite this, the popular perception remained that extra-nuptial pregnancy was still associated with the lower classes as it had been in previous decades. Furthermore it was proposed that "were it not for the reform of abortion laws [and, I suggest, the contraceptive pill], the proportion of illegitimate births to women from the upper social classes would have increased even further" (Gill, 1977, p. 245).

It was challenging for society to accept that middle-class girls became pregnant because they were sexually active:

> It was just too much for the middle-class commentators to accept that a substantial proportion of the population was operating with a code of sexual behaviour antithetical to, if not in direct opposition to that of the value system of the dominant middle class. (Gill, 1977, p. 301)

Not only were unmarried mothers silenced through stigma and shame, but their voices were heard in medical and social discourses only through the filtered, objectified, and predigested accounts of their experiences by psychiatrists, psychologists, and social workers. Consequently, only one side of the adoption story was heard, thereby conveying the impression that mothers surrendered their babies willingly. The stories of coercion and duplicity which would be heard in the 1980s and beyond were absent from previous medical and social discourses.

As an explanation for the decline in white women surrendering their babies from the late 1960s onward in the United States, and from the 1970s in Australia, Grow suggests that "unwed women during this later period may have been subject to less social pressure" (1979, p. 365). If, as Grow claims, "neither social deviancy nor the psychological explanations of the previous era adequately explains why some of the pregnant unwed women of this decade decide to keep and others decide to surrender," then some other explanation had to be proffered (p. 371). I contend that mothers whose babies were considered more desirable were also those more easily persuaded of adoption's social cleansing effects. The unmarried mother, discursively constructed along race and class lines (Solinger, 1994), could be reintegrated in society without a baby as evidence of her moral infraction.

READING KRISTEVA

Julia Kristeva[3] is considered one of the originators of what is known as the French school of postmodern feminism, succeeding Simone de Beauvoir (Grosz, 1989). As Kristeva's theorizing tends toward inaccessibility, clarification of some of her concepts is a valuable precursor to any analysis based on her work. This section offers my understanding of the concepts of the symbolic order, the semiotic order, and abjection, as well as an interpretation of her theory of maternity as it informs mothers' experience of the loss of a baby to adoption.

My reading of Kristeva's work is that the *symbolic order* is the dominant social order that constructs and influences all its social institutions including the family and the law. The symbolic order controls its members through various apparatuses of knowledge, such as the media and popular culture, by constructing the normal and, hence by negation, the deviant and the abject.

The symbolic order renders women invisible and their voices inaudible through objectification in the politicolegal, historical, medical, social, and media discourses on adoption. These discourses privilege certain knowledges, positions, and speakers over others. Privileged discourses assume a scientific, rational position and subjugate other discourses such as those located within the personal. In this way, subjugated or counterhegemonic discourses are stifled and rendered speechless. Within the symbolic, the only socially recognized, validated position for a woman is as a mother (Grosz, 1989).

Whereas the symbolic order can be identified with the social order, the *semiotic order* always operates from the multiple positions of the speaking subject. That is, the semiotic is located within the personal but dissects the social order and its practices, including discourses, constructed within and by it. Kristeva describes the symbolic and semiotic orders as a "permanent contradiction," which instead of occupying conflicting spaces, reinforce each other (1980, p. 139). Likewise the *discourses* of the symbolic and the semiotic confront and yet reinforce each other: the symbolic becomes an order superimposed on the semiotic.

According to Kristeva, the semiotic sits at the borders or the margins of the symbolic from which it threatens and challenges through the speaking subject and through abjection. The speaking subjects are the mothers who lost babies to adoption and the semiotic lies within the counterdiscourses of those speaking, where the counterdiscourses are recognized as legitimate discourses in their own right. The semiotic is also the site of drives and instincts, including the maternal instinct. This relationship is explained further by Kristeva's theory of maternity and the maternal chora (as cited in Moi, 1986).

It is within this model of maternity and motherhood that I examine the meaning of motherhood for women whose babies were taken for adoption. According to Kristeva, the pregnant woman is a manifestation of a split body, a split between "the immeasurable, unconfinable maternal body," which is a "continuous separation, a division of the very flesh" and the maternal chora: the "abyss between the mother and the child" (as cited in Moi, 1986, p. 175). What has been previously part of her own flesh before the birth is "henceforth but irreparably alien" and "irremediably 'an other,'" an alterity between mother and child, posing the questions: Who is the subject? Who is the Other?

My interpretation of Kristeva's notion of the *maternal chora* is that of a spiritual space between the mother and child—a space that *defies* physical boundaries and yet incorporates them; a space that is infinite, that each *defines* in order to become the Other. It is an unreal space, a virtual space, a space that women who have never had children occupy by virtue of their having been daughters. It transcends gender and generations in a metaphysical sense but it is not the biological determinist, maternal instinct. Kristeva is proposing a dialectic between the mother and child across the imposed separation of birth: neither is subject nor object. The taking of a baby for adoption is a rupture in the maternal chora.

Kristeva's work draws together the margins of the symbolic and the semiotic orders at which she sites her theory of abjection, that is, the unnameable and the unspeakable. Kristeva (1982) argues that it is not possible to define *abjection,* for attempting to do so would be situating it within the symbolic: that is, to impose an artificial structure on something fluid and amorphous and which takes on the shape of the abject. Instead, the meaning of abjection can be revealed through metaphor and allegory. For Kristeva "abjection is that which disturbs identity, system and order" and which "exerts greater control if it remains hidden, unknown" (as cited in Lechte, 1990, p. 158).

Kelly Oliver interprets the abject as "something repulsive that both attracts and repels. It holds you there in spite of your disgust. It fascinates . . . The abject is what is on the border, what doesn't respect borders. It is 'ambiguous,' 'in-between,' 'composite'" (1993, p. 55). Oliver goes on to suggest that the symbolic order contains abjection through a system of ritual exclusions (1993). Such exclusion serves to punish moral infractions that pose a "threatening otherness" to the symbolic order (Kristeva, 1982, p. 17). The abject exerts an attraction that "draws me toward the place where meaning collapses" (1982, p. 2) and is therefore a "kind of narcissistic crisis" (1982, p. 14), similar to the crisis of identity that is called up by maternity (as cited in Oliver, 1993).

Kristeva captures the essence of abjection when she theorizes it as "immoral, sinister, scheming, and shady: a terror that dissembles, a hatred that smiles, a passion that uses the body for barter instead of inflaming it, a debtor who sells you up, a friend who stabs you" (1982, p. 4). For many mothers who lost their babies to adoption, abjection is synonymous with adoption.

ADOPTION AS ABJECTION: THE UNNAMEABLE, THE UNSPEAKABLE

Until the 1990s, women who lost babies to adoption were reluctant to speak about their experience openly and without anonymity. Either they spoke under pseudonyms (for example, Inglis, 1984) or their stories were recounted by others. Poised between the dual paradoxes of shame and respectability, they kept their secrets from their families and friends, to themselves and often from themselves. They tried to do what they had been exhorted at the time of their babies' births: pretend the event had never happened, put it behind them, and get on with their lives. One mother, Carol, was advised:

> When I went home I was sort of patted on the head and told to put it all behind me. Never once has my family spoken about this. So . . . it was sort of out, down there with all the other memories, and forgotten.

These women were afraid to speak out because of the disruptions that their disclosure might cause to their present and past families, and to the children whom they had lost. They carried the secret of the loss of their babies alone and in silence, and thought that their experiences were solitary and unimportant. Carol explains:

> It was the shame and the guilt that was put on us by everybody that was so horrendous, and of course it was a big secret and I was never game to talk to, tell anyone about it.

Anne, too, has difficulty talking about the loss of her baby:

> I have had trouble with saying I had a child that I gave up for adoption. It is so hard to get those two sentences out after carrying that secret for eighteen years. It's so hard. I'm very articulate; it's just getting those words out. Because you're expecting that people will judge you more than at the time when you had your baby. Society has moved on, and yet I'm stuck back there with those attitudes. It's terrible.

Mothers whose voices were previously suppressed began speaking up and out about their own pain, the pain of their families, and the iniquities of adoption.

> JACKIE: In a way you're forever branded by something that wasn't your choice, wasn't your fault. I make no bones about it now. I don't hide the fact that I have a daughter and I gave her up for adoption. Sometimes it's not always easy to say, but I don't hide the fact. I don't look to be protected from it, but I do still sometimes feel guilt, because I know that she has abandonment issues, and the guilt I feel is not at giving her up in that regard at all. But I do feel guilty about not having fought for her, and not having fought for me, because nobody ever asked me. I didn't want to give her up; I didn't want to ever give her up. And as you can see, thirty years don't dull it much, do they?

LEE: Well, I feel ashamed in that it is something that is inexcusable on one level, and the thing that really made me feel ashamed was that I had a choice in the matter, but now looking back, I know you didn't have a choice. I still feel guilt, because I don't think that's excusable to abandon your child.

KRISTEN: Why did I allow myself to be stripped of my baby so shockingly? Allow myself to become another bit of adoption fodder? It was all basically to avoid a scandal. The whole thing was pure tragedy—tragedy in its truest meaning occurred because of some flaw in human nature.

In addition to the self-recrimination that Kristen expresses, Lee describes the protracted nature of the grief of her loss beginning at the time of her baby's birth throughout the ensuing years. Her grief seemed to intensify during family celebrations because the source of her grief—her lost child—could not be openly acknowledged:

This grief doesn't start [stop] with perinatal time. It goes on. It goes on when your girlfriends get married and have babies, and you have to break the relationship because you can't stand the sight of their child—you like the child but you just can't stand the sight of the happy family situation. All your sisters get married and have big weddings, or your sister has a cot death [SIDS], and it's the world's biggest tragedy. But what happened to you is nothing. It seems to go on forever. These things happen, and your brothers and sisters have these children and they have their children's birthdays, and you can see the joy they get out of it. I can't cut myself off from my family.

Denise married her baby's father and together they had two daughters. Although she felt that she was living "a reasonably normal life," her pain and feelings of loss continued:

I had hoped that having more children would lessen the feelings of loss for my son, but it did not. I always thought of my son and what he would be doing, particularly on his birthday. I couldn't even send him a birthday card. Sometimes I felt panicky, like I *had* to find him or have some news about him or I would die. I rarely mentioned this to anyone; it made them feel uncomfortable.

Twenty-five years passed before another woman, Kerry, and her mother were able to talk about the adoption. As a result of sharing their secret, Kerry found the will to search for her daughter.

Abjection In/As Birthing

Frida Kahlo's painting titled "My Birth," (as cited in Zamora, 1990) depicts a scene that is familiar to women whose babies were taken for adoption at birth. A woman is giving birth, her head entwined in a sheet; the emerging baby bears the unmistakable facial features of the artist.

ROBYN: I had a pillow held in front of my face when she was born. I remember fighting to get it away but two nurses held it tight while my baby was taken away.

JACKIE: Toward the end they put my legs up in stirrups and I was lying flat on my back and they put a sheet up over my legs so I couldn't see anything or anybody, and they'd just call out to me from behind the screen.

Julie's experience resembles another aspect of this painting: the birthing woman is alone, except for the religious iconography above her bed. This symbol is a reminder of a Christian morality where the cleavage of woman is simultaneously Madonna and whore.

Everybody left the room and they just left me lying there on the delivery table. I don't know how long I was left there on my own.

Kahlo's painting is a metaphor for abjection and relinquishment, rendering the mother invisible and at the same time permitting her to rebirth and get on with her life—advice these mothers frequently heard. As a creative force, Kristeva (1984) compares art with rebirth. Extending this metaphor, Kahlo's painting visually reinforces Kristeva's (1982, p. 3) words: "During that course in which 'I' become, I give birth to myself amid the violence of sobs and vomit."

The mothers whose babies were lost to adoption shortly after birth recount, with varying degrees of horror, their maternity experiences:

JACKIE: I had no idea what was going to happen, what the process was. I'd never heard anyone talk about childbirth or labour. I just had no idea. I was so petrified. Eventually the labour pains became more and more intense and I went into full labour and I went through a dreadful night and the next day dawned and I thought I just couldn't keep going. It was just dreadful. I felt like I had been half out of my mind and half out of my body for days, endlessly, on and on, like floating on top of an ocean. Like I'd ride over the top of the pains when they came, just throw myself right out of my body.

ROBYN: I was so frightened. I didn't have a clue what was going to happen to me. At first I was put into a very large ward with only curtains between the beds. I remember lying there listening to mothers giving birth. Then I must have slept for a while and woke up screaming in pain.

KRISTEN: I had no idea what to expect. The terrifying ordeal had begun. It was like being beside the execution yard. You could hear the victims screaming. I wonder if prisoners on death row feel the same way when the due date of execution comes. I know how torture victims feel—the apprehension, the fear. It was a living, horrible nightmare.

JULIE: Nobody had told me what happens, or what to expect. . . . I went into the delivery room where I was completely and roughly shaved. I remember lying on the table in the delivery room. The baby must have been coming quite fast as they gave me an injection in the vaginal area and then didn't wait for it to take effect. They cut me and I let out a scream.

Referring to abjection, Kristeva writes of the "land of oblivion . . . that is constantly remembered . . . [the] once upon blotted-out time . . . the ashes of oblivion [that] now serve as a screen and reflect aversion, repugnance" (1982, p. 8). Jackie, unable to remember some of the birth events, reflects Kristeva's words:

Nobody would come and speak to me and then the social workers came and I had to sign some things. I don't remember what they were. They assumed that I was going to give my child up for adoption. I don't remember telling anyone—maybe I did, but it's funny, I don't have any memory of saying the words.

"One does not give birth *in* pain, one gives birth *to* pain," says Kristeva (as cited in Moi, 1986, p. 167). For mothers such as Jackie, the pain of childbirth assists them to preserve their sense of self as mother:

I pushed and pushed and pushed and then finally the last push was just dreadful, the pain was so great I lost consciousness. I remember beginning to push and then I don't remember anything else until I came to.

The birth experience has been shrouded in secrecy and shame for these mothers. The joyousness accorded to many women is denied mothers who lose their babies to adoption. Kristen's words capture this experience:

Relinquishment cannot be seen as an isolated complete episode, but as a negative force which continues to affect one's whole life in a most detrimental way.

Many birthing women know that at the end of their travail there will be the long-awaited, hoped-for baby: their labor is a labor of love. For the mothers whose babies were taken for adoption, the pain of their labor has continued, without the joyous resolution that giving birth to a baby should bring them. Barbara recounted the ongoing feelings in this way:

Without warning, the return of the terror and incapacitating pain of loss would overwhelm me. At these moments, the idea of a living but irrevocably lost child triggered the terror experienced during the actual relinquishment.

Abject to Her Baby

For the mother who loses her baby to adoption, her child remains forever a baby, within what I have termed a "pre-Oedipal space." For those mothers who had the opportunity to see their babies, their memories were limited to the early days of their babies' lives.

Denise: He was wrapped up so I couldn't check if he was okay. I could only see his head and hands. He looked so peaceful and I remember thinking how beautiful he was. I reached out to touch his face, and managed to before the sister whisked him away. I never held or saw him again until he turned nineteen.

When Kerry asked to see her baby, her initial request was denied. When she protested, she was allowed to see her newborn for a brief moment:

I was finally allowed to see my baby for about two minutes from a distance of about fifteen feet. The door to my room opened and a nurse stood in the hallway. She held up a bundle with a tiny face peeking out, and then she leaned forward to pull my door closed. I asked her to stop, and asked that she undo the blankets so that I could see for myself that my daughter was okay and "all there." The nurse, obviously reluctant, did as I asked. She unwrapped my baby so that I could have a quick scan. And then the nurse shut the door and was gone.

Cheryl was not only denied the right to see her baby but also denied the right to information:

When I had the baby I was not allowed to see it! Was not informed if it was a boy or girl, no weight, or any information. I asked a sister what weight my baby was and she replied, "You have no right to ask." I only knew she didn't die.

Kristen knew only that she had given birth to a daughter.

The nurses told me that the baby was a girl but there was no other reference to the baby during my hospital stay.

Julie recalls that the only reason she knew that she had given birth to a son was because the staff mentioned this as they recorded the time of the birth:

I did sneak down to the nursery once to see if I could see my baby. Nobody came to talk to me about what was happening. I named him John. I went back again and a nurse was feeding him and she said he was not very well and they didn't tell me what was wrong with him or let me hold him.

From the early days after the adoption throughout the lives of their children, mothers searched for their lost babies.

CHERYL: Anyone in the street with a baby, I struck up a conversation with to find out if it was a boy or a girl, its age, or if the baby was adopted. It's a wonder I wasn't arrested! But gradually I got over it. All I remember of her was her hair as they took her away and I said goodbye.

JACKIE: I would look at every red-headed kid that I ever saw in the street, that would be about the right age, any little girl, and always in the back of my mind was—you never know, miracles might happen—I might find out where she was. And I never stopped fantasising about it.

Denise found employment close to the suburb where her son had been taken, although this meant traveling from one side of the city to the other:

The travelling was onerous but I didn't care if it meant that I might catch a glimpse of him. Every woman with a new baby was the subject of my intense interest. I knew I was acting strangely but I could not behave any other way at that time. I felt jealous of pregnant women because at least they still had their babies with them.

The stages of their babies' development are absorbed into the lives of others, rendering chronologically impossible adoptive parents' fear that the mothers of their children would one day return to reclaim their babies. Many mothers find images of babyhood alienating and too painful to contemplate. These images reinforce their positions as abject mothers—mothers who were not, and are still not, there. The search for their lost children is reflected in Kristeva's words: "Abjection breaks out only when driven to distraction by a desire to know" (1982, p. 83). Kerry thought about her daughter on a regular basis. Instead of her thoughts diminishing over time, they became more frequent:

> I kept my maiden name and made sure that I was listed in the phone book. I thought about her more and more, thought about how I would feel and what I'd say to her and so on. I didn't "consciously" make myself available or start preparing for her return, but I can now see that I *was* getting ready.

Some mothers think of their babies more intensely at certain times of the year:

> CHERYL: Every birthday I would be upset for days before, and I would light a candle and blow it out after I had said, "Happy birthday." Over the years I often wondered, naturally, what she was like. My other daughter begged me for a sister. *Oh God,* I wondered, *what would she say if she knew?*

> ROBYN: Every birthday, every Christmas, I would wonder where she was and what her day was like and if she was being treated well.

Mother's Day is a particularly difficult time for most of these mothers. One mother posted a message of empathy to the other women on the Internet support group. "Hope you all made it through Mother's Day OK. It made me think. Adoption isn't death, but it's just as irreversible." Brenda's poignant response, which she calls "Birthmother Reality," was endorsed unequivocally by the Internet support group:

> Our babies are gone . . . and we know nothing of their baby-ness. Our arms are forever empty of their warmth, their tiny movements. We will never know the tug of their strong little mouths on our breasts, nor the pain of letting the milk come down into their mouths. We will not feel their naked skin next to ours. We will not know the soft downiness of their back, not the fineness of their hair, nor the perfectness of their tiny fingers. We will never see the openness of their stares studying our faces, the first faces they are ever to see. We will never know their cries. We will never know their smell. Our babies no longer exist.

Our children are gone forever . . . and we know nothing of their world. We did not know their friends or their fears. We did not know the names of their favourite stuffed animal, the one they slept with each night. We never heard them cry, "Mummy, I'm scared!" as they go for their immunization. We never did, and we never can . . . those times are irretrievably gone. Our toddlers, our children no longer exist.

Our teenagers with their Sturm und Drang[4] and their puppy loves and the best friend that just told them off are lost to us too. They are gone . . . they belong to the past, and they could not return to us if they wanted to.

Abjection In/As Reunion

Some of the mothers had been reunited with their adopted-away babies, now adults. In many cases the reunions have been joyous, as Kerry recounted:

The best thing that ever happened to me was meeting my daughter. My reunion with her changed my life [for the better] forever. I went through some really tough times in the months just after the reunion. Dealing with all the old stuff that started surfacing after the reunion was not fun. But no matter how uncomfortable or painful things might have been at times, it was worth it. I have my daughter back in my life and nothing could ever be as wonderful, satisfying, and healing as that. . . . Nothing!

However, in other cases, the mother's marginalization from her child's life was reinforced by the discovery of a contact veto: although she received information about her child, she was prohibited legally from making contact with the threat of imprisonment. Anne recounts a mixture of disappointment and disbelief:

I just made a tentative inquiry one day and I was really nervous about it. And when they came back and said there was a contact veto, I just didn't . . . She's twenty-two now. Twenty-three this year.

Lee received a frosty reception from the adoptive parents of her son, James. She was bitterly disappointed that although he had been well provided for materially his upbringing lacked emotional warmth:

When I went to meet my son's adoptive parents she [the adoptive mother] said, "Well his father was disappointed because James is not interested in the things he's interested in." And I thought, *Do you want your money back?* I thought, *This is* my *son you're talking about.* Why would he have the same interests as this man who's not related to him by any sorts of imagination? My son became a disappointment. My precious son. And he's been second best all his life.

Following the birth of her first daughter, Sarah, Cheryl married and had another daughter, Rebecca (Sarah's half-sister). Although Cheryl's reunion with Sarah began propitiously, their relationship deteriorated over a four-year period:

She visited us every couple of months and she and Rebecca became very close. I told her everything she wanted to know. I was so honest: I gave her information sheets from the hospital records and photos of my kids from when they were little to make her feel part of the family.

When she was planning her wedding, Sarah asked Rebecca and her two small daughters to be part of her bridal party. Cheryl was also invited to the wedding, but she declined as "it would have been too hard" to explain her appearance. However, after the wedding Sarah terminated contact. As Cheryl admitted, it was not so much Sarah's rejection of her as the rejection of Rebecca and her daughters who had become close to Sarah. Reunion with the lost child has not provided a panacea to the mother's loss. Instead, it has intensified her loss and reinforced a mother's position as the abject mother.

CHERYL: I just have to wonder why I had to go through it all again only to lose her a second time, but this time hurting others! I just have to wonder whether it was worth it as I envisaged a lot happier times for us all.

In spite of the joyful reunion stories that appear in the media, a subtext remains that the happy stories and the photographs in the media belie. Although many mothers are stuck in a pre-Oedipal space with their infant children, the reality is that when a reunion is effected, mothers find an adult who has been shaped by her or his social circumstances. Mother and adult-child are intimate strangers. Their lives are interwoven as in a helix, touching only at certain points where the pain of adoption and relinquishment recedes to permit a connection. Outside that connection lies abjection where a mother and her child are at the margins. A poem submitted by Lori to the Internet support group articulates these feelings:

> But they did NOT welcome her,
> would not even acknowledge her,
> would not even grant her—
> her humanity.
> She was—and is—the "other" mother.
> She did not know she was not allowed to love him,
> not allowed to care, not allowed to BE.

A nuclear family, such as that demanded of and created by adoption, has room for only one mother. This positioning is most acutely felt and expressed by Cheryl, the abject "other" mother, at family celebrations such as weddings and Christmas:

> Her adoptive mother let me arrange for the wedding cake to be made. It cost $200 but they still thought it only good enough to invite me to the church. I could have been a "friend of the family" at the wedding but they had their own friends there, and didn't want anyone to know that Sarah had gone looking for her "other" family.

Nonetheless, even where mothers are rejected by their now adult children, they feel no hostility—only sadness in the reunion that reinforces abjection. Reunion becomes abjection when understood through Kristeva's words whereby abjection is "something rejected from which one does not part, from which one does not protect oneself" (1982, p. 4). Cheryl's words elaborate further:

> I gave her birthday presents, Christmas presents, invited her and her husband . . . I could go on and on. You can imagine how hard it was for me when I got her "Dear John" letter to say that she felt guilty about coming to us for Christmas and visits when she had her own family.

Kristeva describes the abject as "the jettisoned object [which] is radically excluded . . . [a]nd yet, from its place of banishment, the abject does not cease challenging its master" (1982, p. 2). In response to this challenge, the mother tries to preserve her private sense of self as "mother," while presenting a projected self an "Other" or nonmother. Abjection is the way in which a woman deals with the horror of relinquishment. By preserving her private inner self as "mother," she is able to incorporate the threat of the abject. In becoming the "other" she attempts to resist the abject's challenge, which if she acknowledges, may annihilate her. Kerry writes:

I began thinking about her more and more when she was about eighteen. I found myself fantasising about her, fantasising that she'd come looking for me, and the fantasies were never happy. They were always scary.

Jackie has not met her daughter but maintains contact by telephone and through letters:

I'm afraid to ring too often, afraid to write too often, so I don't. She calls me "Jacqueline"; she sounds like she's talking to her child rather than her mother. She often has a somewhat disapproving tone, and even though I look forward to the possibilities for the future, I'm just going to hang in there and one day she'll be able to acknowledge me for who I really am.

In Australia, when children are taken for adoption at birth, the child's name is recorded as "Unnamed male" or "Unnamed female" with the mother's surname; no father's name is recorded on the birth certificate. In this context, the adopted-away baby can be interpreted as the abject, and qualified only in terms of opposition to the subjective mother.

Following adoption of the baby and its concomitant change in identity, from the unnamed to the nameable, the mother becomes the "jettisoned object," the "abject," an object of defilement, and is perceived as the threat. Where the child was an "other," now the mother without a child becomes the referent, that is, the "other": abjection resides in the ambiguity of the childless mother.

Above all, says Kristeva, abjection is ambiguity. In the "immemorial violence with which the body becomes separated from another body in order to be" (Kristeva, 1982, p. 10) when a woman gives birth to a child, her identity changes irrevocably. In obstetrical terms she is no longer nulliparous and her parity is difficult to conceal subsequently. In social terms, she is a mother since she has borne a child but her reality will never be the same as it was before the birth. Mothers have tried to incorporate this duality whereby "some split themselves into a 'public' side that reunited with society, conformed and did everything acceptably, and a 'private' side that hid, grieved, and felt unworthy" (Jones, 1993, p. 40).

In relinquishment and adoption, abjection preserves a private self as "mother" within the semiotic and a public self within the symbolic. In relinquishment and adoption, maternity is a process with neither subject—"mother"—nor object—"baby": it is abjection.

In the intervening years, some mothers came to realize that they lost their babies permanently because circumstances might not have enabled them to provide for their babies even temporarily.

LEE: You've just got to meet someone to give you a bit support for six months, and then you're on your feet, aren't you?

The mothers' voices through their narratives reveal similar experiences. Each mother's voice blends into the next, like a cacophony of wailing: when one voice subsides as her memories fade, another rises in crescendo to take up the chorus. Repeatedly, mothers tell of how they did not want to surrender their babies, yet through subtly coercive measures, they were seduced into believing that they had no other choice.

The experience of having a baby taken for adoption, while at once unique, has universal qualities across many Western societies, a universality that is unacknowledged. In the primary accounts in this chapter, and in numerous secondary accounts (see, for example, Harkness, 1991; Inglis, 1984; Jones, 1993; Petrie, 1998), mothers' stories share a chilling synchronicity. Without exception, these mothers who are white and middle-class produced babies that were the most prized for the adoption market (Solinger, 1994).

Abject Mothers

For the mothers, writing their stories was consistent with what Kristeva refers to as a "semiotic practice that facilitates the ultimate reorganization of psychic space" (1990, p. 10). Furthermore, the French feminist Hélène Cixous believes that only by writing her individual story can a woman "return to the body which has been more than confiscated from her" (1981, p. 250). Writing their narratives enabled these mothers to do just that, and heal their "psychic space." Some mothers, however, found that it was necessary for them to experience the pain of a reopened wound before the healing began. Without exception, every mother's story contained references to pain and the unhealed wound:

DENISE: It seems true that the pain never really goes away. It just changes.

KRISTEN: The wound is not healed. There is no real cure for this hurt. It has become a familiar emotional lump, lodged somewhere in my brain. I live now with the tears very close under the surface. It is still very raw. It has become part of me, part of my mental baggage. It never goes away. The hurt was so deep, the wound so primal.

SARAH: At this time I have found a certain intellectual or emotional distance from the pain—I don't seem to feel it so much (perhaps it is only numbness?) or perhaps it is that I am learning to stand back from it and observe it rather than being merged with it. Still I am well aware that this grief is not yet dead, only more effectively managed.

LEE: I was having a nervous breakdown basically from the age twenty-two onwards. I was really traumatised by what happened to me. That incident wrecked my life.

JACKIE: And for that month afterwards, and for all the endless months, there's this awful, awful aching pain that doesn't seem to go away. For years and years and years.

CAROL: This'll go on forever. You go away and think about something and come back again. After listening to my story on tape I had a really good cry. It's like in the listening, there's someone else's voice, and how dead it was and the pain that was in it. Incredible. So we still have a lot more pain to get rid of.

KERRY: I didn't feel ordinary. I felt old, different, damaged. My heart grew colder and the wall between myself and other people grew thicker and higher.

MARY: Even though I have continued to live and bulld my wall tall and strong, I will never be whole again.

ROBYN: I have always felt so alone in my anguish and my grief at losing my baby.

For the woman who has lost her baby to adoption, abjection is a result of the permanent ambiguity of the parts she plays either as a nulliparous woman or as a mother, without her being aware of the ambiguity of playing these contradictory roles even when she is consciously aware of acting them out. The mother's "other" self continues to reside in the symbolic order into which the semiotic tries to intervene and subvert. Barbara expressed her sense of ambiguity thus:

> With the passage of time, the intensity of the pain dissipated somewhat, and my emotional life attempted to reestablish itself. Unexpectedly, reminders of my lost child would confront me from without, causing more trauma.

Kristeva's model of maternity as a "process without a subject" (Grosz, 1989, p. 79) assumes a greater "immoral sinister, scheming, shady" tone of abjection (Kristeva, 1982, p. 4). The abjection demanded by adoption for the relinquishment of motherhood is another split between mother and baby superimposed on the separation by birth. In this way Kristeva's notion of abjection is interwoven with her notion of maternity as a process without a subject. In relinquishment and adoption, maternity is a process with neither subject nor object: it is abjection.

REFLECTING ON ABJECTION

The experiences of the mothers recounted in this chapter mirror my own. During the seven years I conducted this research, I have come full circle: from the abject mother who lost her first child to adoption, found him, and was searching for her second, to a re-abjected mother who lost them both yet again. My reunions with my children were very public. In the ecstasy of our reunions we were seduced by print and electronic media to share the joy of our success. I believed that my story was different from those of the other mothers that appear in this chapter. I believed that my children and I would, after our reunion, no longer be abject to each other. This was not the case.

My beliefs were located within the fantasies to which I had clung for more than thirty years. My son wrote to me that he wishes no further contact and has not responded to my correspondence. Neither was I informed of nor invited to my daughter's wedding. She has recently given birth to a son, my first grandchild, but I am not recognized as his grandmother across generations. Like the other women whose voices are heard in this chapter, I remain an abject mother.

NOTES

1. 204,637 between 1960 and 1984 (Annual Adoption Figures, England and Wales, 2001)

2. There are a few notable exceptions. Kate Inglis's "Living Mistakes" (1984) gives voice to sixteen Australian women speaking out about the stigma of extra-nuptial pregnancy and adoption. Anne Petrie's "Gone to an Aunt's" (1998) is a moving account of the stories of seven Canadian women who lost their babies to adoption between 1950 and 1970 with "the promise of salvation that could come only through work and prayer."

3. The title of this section draws from the title of Kelly Oliver's interpretation of Julia Kristeva's theoretical writings.

4. Literally "storm and stress." Refers to a movement of young German writers c. 1770-1782, "characterised by passion and energetic repudiation of the rules of French critics" (Little, Fowler, & Couslon, 1992, p. 2139).

REFERENCES

Annual adoption figures, England and Wales 1960-1984. (2001). 1960-1973: Her Majesty's Stationery Office, Registrar General's Statistical Review of England and Wales, Table T5; OPCS Monitor, Table 3. <http://www.plumsite.com/abortion>.

Atwood, M. (1987). *The handmaid's tale.* London: Virago

Carangelo, R. (2004). Statistics of adoption. <http://www.kearan.com/lori/statistics.html>.

Cixous, H. (1981). The laugh of the Medusa. In E. Marks, & I. de Coutivron (Eds.), *New French feminisms: An anthology* (pp. 240-263). New York: Harvester Wheatsheaf.

Derdeyn, A.P. & Wadlington,W.J. (1977). Adoption: The rights of the parents versus the best interests of their children. *Journal of the American Academy of Child Psychiatry, 16*(2), 238-255.

Farrar, P.D. (1997). *An annotated directory of adoption and related literature.* New South Wales Department of Community Services, Sydney, Australia.

Farrar, P.D. (2000). Relinquishment and abjection: A semanalysis of the meaning of losing a baby to adoption. Unpublished doctoral dissertation, University of Technology, Sydney, Australia.

Gill, D. (1977). *Illegitimacy, sexuality and the status of women.* Oxford, UK: Basil Blackwell.

Goldstein, J., Freud, A., & Solnit, A.J. (1973). *Beyond the best interests of the child.* New York: Free Press.

Grosz, E. (1989). *Sexual subversions: Three French feminists.* Sydney: Allen and Unwin.

Grow, L.J. (1979). Today's unmarried mothers: The choices have changed. *Child Welfare, 58*(6), 363-371.

Harkness, L. (1991). *Looking for Lisa.* Sydney: Random House.

Inglis, K. (1984). *Living mistakes: Mothers who consented to adoption.* Sydney: George Allen and Unwin.

Jones, M.B. (1993). *Birthmothers: Women who have relinquished babies for adoption.* Chicago: Chicago Review Press.

Kristeva, J. (1980). *Desire in language: A semiotic approach to literature and art.* New York: Columbia University Press.

Kristeva, J. (1982). *Powers of horror: An essay on abjection.* New York: Columbia University Press.

Kristeva, J. (1984). *Revolution in poetic language.* New York: Columbia University Press.

Kristeva, J. (1990). The adolescent novel. In J. Fletcher & A. Benjamin (Eds.), *Abjection, melancholia and love: The work of Julia Kristeva* (pp. 1-22). London: Routledge.

Lechte, J. (1990). *Julia Kristeva.* London: Routledge.

Little, W., Fowler, H.W., & Coulson, J. (1992). *Shorter Oxford English Dictionary (OED)* (3rd Ed.). Oxford: Clarendon Press.

Moi, T. (Ed.). (1986). *The Kristeva reader.* Oxford: Basil Blackwell.

Oliver, K. (1993). *Reading Kristeva: Unraveling the double-bind.* Bloomington: Indiana University Press.

Petrie, Anne. (1998). *Gone to an aunt's: Remembering Canada's homes for unwed mothers.* Toronto: McClelland and Stewart.

Rains, P.M. (1970). Moral reinstatement: The characteristics of maternity homes. *American Behavioral Scientist, 14*(2), 219-235.

Solinger, R. (1994). *Wake up little Susie: Single pregnancy and race before Roe v. Wade.* New York: Routledge.

Zamora, M. (1990). *Frida Kahlo: The brush of anguish.* Seattle: Art Data.

Chapter 4

Clarifying Choice:
Identity, Trauma, and Motherhood

Linda L. Anderson

Imagine a young woman who likes to play volleyball, fish in a clean river, photograph sunsets, and construct fabric teddy bears. Intelligent, committed, active, and dedicated to her own personal growth, she can appreciate camping in the woods as keenly as she can empathize with her clients recovering from drug abuse. Imagine this same woman carrying around a painful secret of choosing to leave her two young children in the care of their father so that she could finally find herself in the chaos of her own life's experience.

Cynthia* is a forty-four-year-old white, middle-class woman who grew up in New Hampshire. She first came to me for counseling citing problems in her lesbian relationship as well as concerns about her clinical depression, her recovery from substance abuse, her sexual identity, and her relationship with her two children. Over time she has been able to resolve many of her conflicts in these various areas, but one extremely difficult area of distress has often been her feelings about being a mother and her bond with her children.

My counseling practice consists primarily of clients such as Cynthia who are survivors of childhood abuse, and I use many different approaches when working with clients. We learned that many of Cynthia's negative and painful feelings surrounding her identity as a mother were intricately connected to the other issues with which she was struggling. Much of our exploration at the beginning of her therapy was about her childhood abuse, and her coming to see the truth of what had happened to her, and the effects it produced in her adult life.

---

*Pseudonyms have been used for all persons.

It seemed to me that interviewing Cynthia about her children, Scott and Elizabeth, and her decision to live apart from them would provide a narrative of interest to others. Moreover, the interview would be of benefit to Cynthia, as it provided another creative way of chipping away at an intransigently negative and destructive pattern of thinking and feeling.

This chapter illuminates how the various emotional struggles Cynthia faced contributed to her decision to live apart from her children. More broadly, this chapter challenges the familiar assumptions that all women are content in the traditional mother role and that staying with one's children no matter what is always the best choice for women and their children. So many powerful elements inform a woman's approach to, perception of, and experience in her role as mother that we cannot automatically make conclusions about the character or ability of the individual woman in that role. Perhaps most important, I want to show therapeutic ways in which a woman can be helped to feel less guilty and ashamed and more empowered by her choices, no matter how the culture has diminished the legitimacy of those choices. By clarifying Cynthia's choice, this work illustrates how living apart from one's own children can be a healthy move for all concerned.

The interview was conducted with Cynthia's full cooperation as an adjunct to our work. I accepted no fee payment for her participation. I subscribe to and maintain strong boundaries with my clients and believe that none were weakened during the preparation of this manuscript. Cynthia read and commented on this manuscript and felt included in decisions about the final work product. Just as I had hoped, the interviewing process and resulting manuscript helped Cynthia more deeply understand her choices and assuage some of her remorse and guilt regarding her role as mother to her children.

The next section presents an edited version of the one-hour taped interview with Cynthia. This is followed by an analysis of the interview within the context of literature on identity, motherhood, and trauma. My intent is to show the ways in which Cynthia's feelings and thoughts are intertwined with her own childhood experiences, her dealings with legal and health professionals, her heterosexual marriage to William, and broader political and cultural realities.

CLARIFYING CHOICE: CYNTHIA'S STORY

LINDA: Tell me the circumstances in which you decided to live apart from your kids, and start from wherever you want.

CYNTHIA: I think the first inkling came when their father and I were discussing divorce. He started crying and said, "Don't take my children away from me." So that was part of the decision. The other part was that I had been a full-time mother for, at that point, three and a half years, and I was just feeling burned out by it. I didn't have any support. My mom had died before Scott was born—that was my first child—and my family wasn't very supportive. So that also played into this decision. The other thing was that I had gotten into recovery. I had been a pothead and couldn't stop. I got into Narcotics Anonymous in March of 1987 and then made this decision [to not live with the kids] about a year later. I relapsed over the decision because part of what played into [it] was me coming out as a lesbian. And I hadn't really had any clue before that, and then it all kind of came together, and I didn't want [being a lesbian] coming out in court to be used against me, and maybe against me as a mother to my children.

LINDA: When your husband said after you asked for a divorce, "Don't take my children away from me," did that make you feel guilty? Had you wanted the kids to live with you or did you want some kind of joint custody? Why do you specifically mention that phrase?

CYNTHIA: Because I wanted joint custody, I hadn't really thought too much about who was going to get them, and how we were going to work that out because that was just the beginning of the process of working it out. It didn't cause me to feel guilty. It actually caused me to feel some relief that I don't have to do it all. Because I had been doing it all pretty much.

LINDA: Can you say more about feeling burned out as a mother, what that means to you?

CYNTHIA: The first thing that comes to mind is remembering how my life revolved around them and that having a dentist appointment to go to was a big deal. Like I was doing something for me. Because I really didn't do much for me. I was just with them all the time and they were twenty-two months apart, so it was tough, having two babies. Actually I think that's what helped me hit bottom, realizing that I needed to stop getting high, because my way of coping with anything was to get high, and having two babies I couldn't do that. Even though I wanted to, even though I tried to.

LINDA: So you weren't working outside the home at all during this time?

CYNTHIA: No.

LINDA: You were with the kids all day long, twenty-four seven.

CYNTHIA: Yep.

LINDA: Did you feel like you were losing yourself?

CYNTHIA: Yes, especially when my husband would call me mommy, and I never got called by my name, or the self became the mommy. That was my identity. To not just him but his parents, who were the children's grandparents.

LINDA: Did you have an identity before you had the kids? A conscious identity that you felt you had to give up?

CYNTHIA: [Long pause.] I know that part of the identity at that point, before the children, was my work. At that point I was doing physical therapy aide work.

LINDA: And you gave that up once you had the children.

CYNTHIA: Right.

LINDA: Did you want to have the children?

CYNTHIA: Yeah.

LINDA: You wanted to be a mom?

CYNTHIA: Yep.

LINDA: How come?

CYNTHIA: I don't know. Sometimes I wonder if it was because I thought that would be the answer, that that would take away my misery.

LINDA: That having children would fix things and make things better, both for you and the marriage?

CYNTHIA: Yeah.

LINDA: Did your husband want children?

CYNTHIA: Yeah.

LINDA: Can you describe to me what it was like to be with them all day long? You said there was no time for you to do the things that you needed for yourself, that everybody called you mommy, and you lost your identity. What was a day with two little toddlers like for you?

CYNTHIA: It was pretty insane. I remember not even being able to use the toilet sometimes. I'd have to literally lock Scott in his room so that he would not attack his sister, so that I could go to the toilet. Or I would take her into the bathroom with me. Cause he was very angry with the fact that I had brought home his sister, even though we had done the preliminary "getting ready for the new baby" thing. But he was number one in his father's eyes.

LINDA: So he was angry at the new baby, and angry at you?

CYNTHIA: Yeah. He didn't talk to me for three months when I brought her home. He was almost two years old.

LINDA: Literally didn't talk to you?

CYNTHIA: Yeah, pretty much.

LINDA: Did he talk to his dad?

CYNTHIA: Yep.

LINDA: How did you feel about him not talking to you? That's pretty dramatic.

CYNTHIA: Well, I knew that it was a period that he had to adjust to. And there were also other changes going on. I had started him in day care during the last months of my pregnancy and continued that after Elizabeth was born. I don't think he was angry about having to go there. But it was a change that he had to adjust to.

LINDA: Did he continue to talk to your husband?

CYNTHIA: I think so.

LINDA. Did you ask for support? Did you know you needed it?

CYNTHIA: Yes, I went to a mothers' support group when Scott was six months old. I broke down in the doctor's office just talking about how I didn't know what was wrong with him, and I think it was teething, or stuff like that, and the doctor referred me to this mothers' support group, and it was very helpful to realize that all mothers felt that way, and it was okay to feel that way, and that it wasn't a bad thing, or unusual, or negative.

LINDA: You were smoking pot throughout this whole time?

CYNTHIA: Yep.

LINDA: You said that at some point you realized that you had to stop that. How old were the kids when you realized you had to stop that?

CYNTHIA: It was right around when Elizabeth was born. Because I had tried to control my use while I was pregnant, but I wasn't able to stop completely. I knew that I needed to have all my wits about me.

LINDA: You needed all your energy. So you got into Narcotics Anonymous [NA]?

CYNTHIA: Yep. I got all set to tell the leader of the mothers' group one day [that I was an addict], and she wasn't there. So I ended up telling the therapist that was there. Eventually the regular group leader referred me to a therapist who I went to two or three times, before she directed me to a women's NA meeting, and I went. And after that I went every day. I didn't know anything about recovery or treatment programs or getting help or anything like that.

LINDA: Did you talk about being a mother in those meetings?

CYNTHIA: Yeah.

LINDA: What was the progression about when you left your husband? How soon after you started NA did you decide to get divorced or separated?

CYNTHIA: About a year later I started getting messages to look at my sexual identity, and I was, so I was having a hard time with it, because I didn't want to be different or ostracized or anything like that.

LINDA: Had your husband been smoking pot while you were in NA?

CYNTHIA: Yeah. But not in front of me. Secretly. Like there was a friend we used to buy pot from who would come over, and she and William would take a walk. And I knew what they were doing but I got pissed off 'cause I couldn't do it too! But that's all part of the recovery thing.

LINDA: And was that part of the marriage breaking down as well?

CYNTHIA: Probably, but not a big part.

LINDA: The biggest part was your sexual identity?

CYNTHIA: Right. The other big part was the disrespect that I felt from him to the point where my son came first. And if I had an opinion about something, like the toys would be all over the living room, and I was trying to teach Scott to pick them up, William would say,

"No, he doesn't need to do that," and he would pick them up himself. This boy did not know how to close doors behind himself because his father did everything for him. Now he's sixteen years old and he still says, "I don't know. I've gotta ask my dad!" [laughter] He's getting better though.

LINDA: So how did you deal with the sexual identity issue. How did you deal with knowing that you were a lesbian?

CYNTHIA: I started talking to the therapist who was the head of the mothers' support group, and it turned out she had had a similar experience but didn't really want me to know, because she was in the closet, so to speak. When I did finally get that information, she really didn't want to have anything to do with me after that. I don't know why. Her stuff.

LINDA: She felt threatened?

CYNTHIA: Maybe. Like I was gonna tell the world. I don't know. So that was part of it. I also was in a meeting one night, and a woman that I knew for a while started talking about herself and dealing with [being gay]. So I approached her, and we made plans to go to a gay NA meeting. So we went. And then I started getting involved in the NA Roundup, the yearly convention, and had my first lesbian relationship in the summer to fall of '89.

LINDA: Had you left William by then?

CYNTHIA: No, I was living in the basement in my own makeshift room from April, and then I left and got my own apartment in October.

LINDA: What were your feelings toward the children at this time?

CYNTHIA: Through the process of getting sober, coming out as a lesbian, going through a divorce? It was just hard for me to switch gears and take care of my own needs more than I had when I was being a full-time mother. I went back to work, got a per diem job in the fall of 1987, but it really wasn't much. And then started working part-time in August of 1988.

LINDA: Who was watching the children when you were working and going to meetings?

CYNTHIA: Their father. He was good about that because I did go to meetings every night, and he had to give them their baths and put them to bed. Sometimes I felt guilty about that, because I wasn't there, but I made it a point to be there a couple nights a week, to do that, because I felt I was missing out on something, even though it was work, it was still being with them.

LINDA: So tell me about when you actually left the house, and made the decision that the children were not going to come with you.

CYNTHIA: Well, we had been to family court to discuss that issue, and it had been agreed on that they were going to stay with their father, and I was going to have visitation. And visitation was only one night a week, for a couple of hours, and every other weekend, and it was left as "or any other time agreed upon by both parties." And there were a couple of times when I stopped by the house to try to see them, and the police were called because he didn't want me to be there. So the first time I left before the police came; the second time I stayed and made him show the police the paperwork, and the police said there really isn't anything they could do. And I said, "Oh, so it was my fault for letting that go through with that wording, knowing that he was going to be an asshole." So my relationship with the kids suffered because it was extra hard and more work to try to see them, to even be a part-time mother to them, and I still had no support, and their father was telling them negative things about me. It was just tough.

LINDA: Tell me about the day you actually left the house knowing that you would only see them one night a week and every other weekend? Do you remember that day?

CYNTHIA: Yeah. I mean it was exciting, because we had been at that point separated for a year anyhow, not a couple.

LINDA: But you were still living in the house.

CYNTHIA: Right.

LINDA: And where were you going to? To your own apartment?

CYNTHIA: Yeah.

LINDA: And how old were the children now?

CYNTHIA: Scott was going on five, and Elizabeth was just three.

LINDA: What did you say to them about what was going to happen?

CYNTHIA: I think I'd been talking about it as time went on. That I would be going to my own place, and they would be coming over to visit with me, and I would like to come and visit with them if their father allowed it, you know. It was going to be up to him. I think they pretty much understood because it had been a process. It wasn't like, boom, all of a sudden I'm going.

LINDA: What were their feelings about you not living at the house anymore?

CYNTHIA: I know my daughter missed me. Scott was tough, because he expressed his anger, and he played off of his father's anger. So it was hard to work out that relationship with him.

LINDA: How do you know your daughter missed you?

CYNTHIA: She would say so, or when she would see me she would get all excited.

LINDA: Was Scott angry at you?

CYNTHIA: Yes.

LINDA: What would he do?

CYNTHIA: Sometimes he would say he didn't want to come when it was visiting time.

LINDA: Would he say why?

CYNTHIA: No.

LINDA: But you knew.

CYNTHIA: Yeah.

LINDA: And how did you feel about their reaction?

CYNTHIA: Bad. Guilty. Feeling that I abandoned them. I almost had to rationalize to myself that I hadn't, because it wasn't okay with me that sometimes I only saw them once a week. I even felt the guilt recently, like a year or two ago, when there was a little girl living next door to us who was three, and that's how old Elizabeth was when I left. [This little girl] would be looking out the window and she would be saying, "My mommy's coming home!" And I thought that Elizabeth was that little, and I wasn't coming home. [Tears.]

LINDA: What makes you cry about it now?

CYNTHIA: Well, I still wish there had been some way to have it more equal, that I could have been able to have them part-time.

LINDA: And why was that not possible?

CYNTHIA: Because their father wasn't willing to work it out.

LINDA: So the agreement with the court was you would see them one night a week and every other weekend. Did William want that arrangement more than you?

CYNTHIA: I don't even remember.

LINDA: But you felt a sense of relief knowing that you would not have to have that responsibility every day?

CYNTHIA: Right.

LINDA: So was it in fact easier on you not to have to take care of them every day?

CYNTHIA: Well, it went back and forth. There was some relief in that, but there was also the missing them, and not being able to see them when I wanted to, or to work things out so that I could feel closer to them.

LINDA: So it was William who made it difficult for you to get more time with them, because even though the court's agreement was that you could see them at any time both of you agreed, he really made it hard for that to happen.

CYNTHIA: Yeah.

LINDA: Did he want the marriage to continue?

CYNTHIA: Yep.

LINDA: So he was punishing you?

CYNTHIA: Yeah, he was angry for years. Probably ten years.

LINDA: So when you talk about feeling guilty, and you have over the years that I've worked with you around this issue, you haven't really gotten to the point of being angry at William for preventing you from having the kind of time you wanted with the children.

CYNTHIA: Yeah, I'm angry with him.

LINDA: But you still take it out on yourself, as guilt, that you have done something bad or wrong.

CYNTHIA: Yeah, 'cause it feels like an excuse. If I don't feel guilty, and I get mad at him about it, then it feels like an excuse for me to feel okay about the whole situation, about leaving the kids, like sometimes feeling I abandoned them, and having to rationalize to myself that I didn't.

LINDA: And the way I see it is that you felt like you were disappearing. You were addicted to pot, you were dealing with your sexual identity, you were not happy in this marriage, and you were overwhelmed by being a mother.

CYNTHIA: Yeah.

LINDA: And the way you wanted to deal with that was to get away from your husband, with whom you didn't want to be any longer, and to share more of the work of raising the kids. That's very different from what happened. And it sounds like you didn't have a lot of control over what happened. Because if you had had your choice, you would have been able to see them more often.

CYNTHIA: Right.

LINDA: So in that scenario that I've just painted, guilt is not the appropriate response because you have in fact done nothing wrong. You were doing what was right for you and ultimately right for the children, and your ex-husband prevented you from having the relationship you wanted with them.

CYNTHIA: Yeah, and that reminds me of how I felt that if I had fought to be the primary caregiver that I would have been angry with [the kids] for having to do that. I felt like I was not taking care of myself and was totally giving my whole life to being a mother, and I didn't want it to affect them in that way.

LINDA: Right. Right. Right. That's an important point. You didn't want to be the primary caregiver any longer, but you did want some kind of equality around caregiving, and you also said you don't remember how the court decision was made.

CYNTHIA: Right.

LINDA: Can you say something about why you don't remember it, or what it means that you don't remember it? Was it out of your control? Was that what William wanted and you didn't feel like you could push against it? Was it what the judge suggested? Do you have any sense of how that came to be? Or did you think that because there was the caveat that you could see the kids whenever you wanted when it was agreeable to both people, that that would cover it, that you didn't anticipate William being as resistant and cruel as he ended up?

CYNTHIA: Yeah, I think that was it, as best I can remember.

LINDA: And I think that he was profoundly cruel to you in that. He was using the children as a pawn, which was not fair to them at all.

CYNTHIA: Yeah. Right. And I remember over the years having tried to discuss with him some way of me being more involved with them, whether it was half the year with me, half the year with him, or so many days a week, this way and that way, we discussed that some, but . . . The children had a therapist that they were going to, and I went in a couple of times because she felt it necessary that Scott deal with his anger toward me. He was resistant to do that. So we never really did that, but I did speak with her about what she thought would be appropriate or good or in their best interest about those kinds of arrangements, here and there, or half and half. Basically it was felt that that wasn't the best arrangement.

LINDA: How come?

CYNTHIA: Because it would be too chaotic for them.

LINDA: Did she know you were a lesbian?

CYNTHIA: Yes.

LINDA: Do you think that figured into her opinion of it at all?

CYNTHIA: Maybe.

LINDA: Why did she say it was too chaotic?

CYNTHIA: Because at that point we were living in different towns, and we would have had to work out the school stuff, and the kids would become confused about where they were going when, and things like that.

LINDA: Even though some people have been able to make those arrangements?

CYNTHIA: I wish that I had had a better lawyer, not just for the divorce, but I wish I had found a good lawyer to help me with that.

LINDA: What age are the kids when the therapist said it would be too chaotic?

CYNTHIA: They were in grade school, it was probably the early nineties, so they were four and six, or six and eight.

LINDA: So what's happened since then?

CYNTHIA: I was laid off in 1996, and that gave me the opportunity to have my daughter spend the summer with us, me and my partner. She had her own room, and she had her own pets, and it was just nice. I took her to the bus to go to day camp, and went to day camp, and did those kinds of things. I did always feel "not a part of" when I did those mother things, like camp stuff or going to school, or things like that, because I wasn't involved in their daily lives. So I always felt left out somehow, and then I felt guilty about that. But William has since eased his anger in the last year or two, and now wants to be friends, and I'm still pissed at him, that jerk, and I need to remember what an asshole and a jerk he was, and it's not hard to remember. And I have documentation I can look at if I need to, to remind me.

LINDA: Talk more about feeling left out as a mother, and what leaving the kids and not being able to see them as much as you wanted to did to your sense of yourself as a mother?

CYNTHIA: Well, my sense of myself was that I was an absentee mother, because I didn't know what my children ate for breakfast. I didn't know what time they went to school. I didn't know sometimes even who their teachers were. And that was the kind of thing I probably could have insisted more on knowing. But in order to be able to do that I would have had to been able to talk with their father on a reasonable level, and that wasn't going to happen.

LINDA: What was it like to try to talk to him about this stuff?

CYNTHIA: He was very withholding and resistant to letting me in on any of that. Once in a while I would be told about maybe an open house at the school or a Thanksgiving skit or program that they might be involved in.

LINDA: But to get any regular kind of information from him was very difficult.

CYNTHIA: Sometimes I wonder if I shouldn't have tried harder. But I didn't really have anywhere to go. I mean, what am I gonna do, go to the school and say "I'm so and so's mother, and they live with their father, and he's a jerk, and I want to know."

LINDA: [I nod that she could have done this.]

CYNTHIA: Yeah, see, I could have, but I didn't. Because I didn't have enough energy to do that.

LINDA: Right. Do you want to talk about your clinical depression?

CYNTHIA: I think I've always been depressed. And my first therapist started suggesting that I consider some antidepressant medication. At that point I had been clean, I don't remember how long, but I wasn't willing to [take medication] because I felt like it was violating my recovery, and she pretty much said I don't think we can go any further unless you do that. So I said, "Okay, bye," and I went and got another therapist.

LINDA: What year was that?

CYNTHIA: I think it was [19]89 or [19]90 when the divorce was going through. And I remember feeling pretty ill one December, and just not up to par, and I went to my medical doctor and he suggested that I try an antidepressant. And that was the third professional in my life [who recommended medication]. The first one was after my mom had died. So I [took the antidepressant], and it helped tremendously. I think it helped me to make that decision to get out of my unhappy marriage.

LINDA: When you got out of the marriage and you were no longer living with the kids, you were able to explore your sexual identity more, get a full-time job?

CYNTHIA: Yep. Went to school and got my bachelor's degree finished.

LINDA: And how did all of those things change you?

CYNTHIA: Well, it gave me the opportunity to get in touch with myself, to be true to myself, to seek what was important to me.

LINDA: And what is your relationship with your kids now?

CYNTHIA: Good! I still see them maybe once, sometimes twice a week. They are fourteen and sixteen, soon to be fifteen and seventeen, and have their own lives, but I find it's been important to them to come on those nights, the night of the week, to be with me. And I'm not sure, I think that they know how difficult it was for me and how I tried to see them more. I talked to them about that. And now that I have multiple sclerosis [MS], I don't know if that plays any part in it or not.

LINDA: In what?

CYNTHIA: In their wanting to see me.

LINDA: What do you mean?

CYNTHIA: Because my partner has said some things, to especially Scott, about coming to see me. I guess she's told them how important it is to me, and he's been honoring that.

LINDA: There was a while when he wasn't coming over, right?

CYNTHIA: Right. He was going through a tough period in his life, and I'm not even sure exactly what it was, but he was nine or ten, and he really just didn't want to come over.

LINDA: How long did that last?

CYNTHIA: A few months, not real long.

LINDA: How did you feel about that, him not wanting to come over?

CYNTHIA: Well, I felt bad, but I didn't turn it on myself so much. I knew it was just something he was going through.

LINDA: But even before you had MS, they wanted to come see you.

CYNTHIA: Right.

LINDA: So that's not the only reason. And you feel like you have a close relationship with them.

CYNTHIA: Yeah.

LINDA: So in hindsight, how do you feel about your decision to live apart from your children?

CYNTHIA: There may have only been a couple of times that I really wished I had made another decision, but generally I feel okay about that. Of course I wish that I could have seen them more or worked things out on a more equal basis, but it was a fight to do what little I did do.

LINDA: And that was the price you ended up paying to hold onto your own self.

CYNTHIA: Yep.

LINDA: And it wasn't your choice. You would have preferred to spend more time with them.

CYNTHIA: Right.

LINDA: I think that's the part that you forget.

CYNTHIA: Yeah, because I have this thing in my head, like, if one of my clients is a mother, and her kids don't live with her, I think, "What's wrong with her?" So I do that to myself, too. What's wrong with me that my kids didn't live with me full-time?

LINDA: And do you still frame it that way, that there was something wrong with you?

CYNTHIA: No, there's just reasons.

LINDA: How did people around you, your friends and family react?

CYNTHIA: Nobody really said anything against it, against the decision. I think some of the family thought it was a little strange that I wasn't more involved in their lives when they were younger.

LINDA: But no one actively criticized you?

CYNTHIA: No.

LINDA: Did William?

CYNTHIA: I don't think to me he did, but I think in front of the children he did. I think that's what made it worse was that, I mean I don't know exactly what it was he was saying to them, but he could have been saying things like, well, your mother left you, or things like that. So it made it all the more difficult for me to not only show them that that's not exactly what happened, but to feel that way for myself.

LINDA: So did you feel for a long time like you had left them or abandoned them?

CYNTHIA: Yeah, in a way, yeah.

LINDA: Rather than just sort of changing over the situation. It sounds like that's what you were trying to do. You weren't trying to leave or abandon them. You were trying to get a break, trying to get some help. You were trying to deal with your depression, your sexual identity, and you were trying to hold onto yourself.

CYNTHIA: Yeah.

LINDA: And spend more time with the kids.

CYNTHIA: Yep.

LINDA: And even though your relationship with them has stayed intact and is a good one, because of William's resistance you missed out on a lot of their growing up, and that's something that's a big source of pain for you.

CYNTHIA: Yeah. I wish there had been some way that it could have been different, or I wonder if I didn't do enough to make it happen.

LINDA: The way I hear this story, my feeling is that you did all that you could do at the time. Meaning whatever time it happened to be, whether it was fifteen years ago, or ten years ago, or eight years ago. That your ability to push for what you wanted and even be clear about what you wanted and needed was difficult for you to do.

CYNTHIA: Yeah, because I was alone in that. I didn't have any support.

LINDA: How do you feel now that we've talked about this?

CYNTHIA: Mixed. Sad, but okay, the way things had to be. Not that I don't wish that some of it were different, but that's the way it was, and that's the way it had to be, and I think it's important to me that they understand that I did what I could. That it wasn't that I didn't want to be a part of their lives.

LINDA: Do you think they understand that now?

CYNTHIA: I hope so. I think probably some.

LINDA: Is that something you want to keep reassuring them about?

CYNTHIA: I'd like to talk with them a little more about it.

LINDA: I think that would be good for all of you to do that. And what's the biggest sadness about this whole part of your life?

CYNTHIA: That whole part? That I was their mother in reality but I didn't feel like their mother a lot of the time.

LINDA: I wonder if part of your sadness is feeling that there's so much pressure from the culture about what kind of mother you were supposed to be, or what kind of mother you are supposed to be now?

CYNTHIA: Yeah, I think so.

LINDA: It sounds like you were trying to define a kind of motherhood that would work for you. It wasn't that you didn't want these children. You wanted to have a relationship with them that allowed you to have yourself as well, and that wasn't happening.

CYNTHIA: Yeah. It almost feels selfish, though, I guess because of the way my mother was. In that she always put herself last, and didn't really think about her own needs or desires, and I believe that's part of why she died of cancer at that young age.

LINDA: How old was she?

CYNTHIA: Fifty-four.

LINDA: Right, we all get our models of what a mother is from our own mothers. And as you said there weren't people helping you to figure out how to do this. It's very common that women get left home with the kids, and you're supposed to do it!

CYNTHIA: But I still feel lucky that I had that opportunity to be a stay-at-home mom, because I think it would have been more work and more trying and more difficult to balance taking care of babies and working.

LINDA: Even if William had picked up half of the load?

CYNTHIA: Well, I don't know . . .

REFLECTIONS ON IDENTITY, MOTHERHOOD, AND TRAUMA

This interview reveals several aspects important to understanding Cynthia's reasons for living apart from her children. She entered her marriage with a history of childhood abuse, an impaired sense of self-worth, and a particular set of parenting models. She experienced substance abuse, addiction, and undiagnosed clinical depression. Her sexual identity was becoming clearer to her at a time when being a lesbian and a mother was a combination discriminated against in a myriad of ways. Cynthia's husband was not supportive, pushing her into the role of selfless, omnipresent motherhood. Although she resisted this role, she had neither extended family, friends, nor community to help her. Turning to professionals for survival, she was again disappointed and given inadequate support for many of her challenges.

Unexpressed in the interview, and one salient and profound part of Cynthia's story, is her history of emotional and physical abuse by her father, and the unprotective stance and general passivity of her mother. Cynthia lived with various levels of post-traumatic stress syndrome (PTSS) throughout her life. Some of the results of PTSS have been her self-medication through drug abuse, loss of memories from large portions of her childhood, inability to advocate for herself in important situations, and the development of clinical depression. Much of her life, Cynthia lived in a state of fear, confusion, and pain. Her remarks in the interview often indicate her lack of clarity on the events surrounding her leaving her children, and an inconsistent response to the same question worded differently.

Judith Herman (1997) defines post-traumatic stress syndrome as that set of wide-ranging symptoms including generalized anxiety, "extreme startle response to unexpected stimuli" (p. 36), inability to tune out repetitive stimuli, difficulty sleeping, noise sensitivity, problems of relatedness and identity, hypervigilance, low self-esteem, somatic complaints, tension, depression, a capacity to "restrict and suppress" (p. 89) thoughts, as well as numerous other characteristics.

Women with PTSS brought on from childhood abuse often become adults ill-equipped to take on the enormous responsibilities of caring for their children. Unless the mother has been able to work through the pain of her own abuse, she is likely to have difficult emotions triggered by the repeated demands of her own children. According to Eliana Gil, many survivors of childhood abuse experience problems in parenting.

> Parenting problems were defined as difficulties in caring for children. Most adults abused as children have not had appropriate modeling regarding discipline and communication with children. They feel at a loss when they themselves become parents. Some . . . were keenly cognizant of the so-called cycle of child abuse. These clients asked for specific help to avoid hurting their own children. They asked to be taught how to show love and affection, while at the same time setting limits. (1988, p. 51)

Because Cynthia was not allowed to express or have met her own normal childhood needs or have those needs validated, it became nearly impossible for her as a mother to respond to her own children's needs without numbing out or experiencing a diminution of her own identity. At that time, she was clearly experiencing many of the elements of PTSS, which would make raising two small children a kind of hell.

Cynthia became pregnant with her first child, Scott, the same year that her mother died. She was grieving her mother throughout the pregnancy and after the birth of her son. Sadness about her mother not being around to see her grandson was painful for her. Losing her mother as well as unresolved feelings of rage and terror from her childhood seriously compromised her ability to tackle the demands of being a young first-time mother. She had learned a great deal about submission and passivity from her mother in relation to enduring abuse from her father.

Cynthia was unprepared for motherhood. As Sheila Kitzinger states:

> Part of the problem is that we have far too little education for parenthood, for either expectant mother or father, but this is not just a question of classes in the weeks before the baby comes. To be effective, preparation for the major life crisis of becoming a

parent has to take place both in adolescence, as part of learning about adult roles, and even earlier, in the prospective parents' own childhood. For many of today's mothers parenthood, however welcome, comes as a surprise. (1980, p. 16)

At best, women with relatively safe and nurturing childhoods are faced with an enormous challenge when becoming a mother. Children from dysfunctional, abusive, and terrifying circumstances can be set up for untold problems when embarking on motherhood. Cynthia had undeveloped coping skills; she was battling drug addiction and undiagnosed clinical depression. Moreover, her own mother was not present in her life to offer the possibility of support, companionship, and nurturance.

Cynthia came into the marriage and motherhood with no clearly defined sense of herself or her identity. Gwyn Kirk and Margo Okazawa-Rey write:

Our identity is a specific marker of how we define ourselves at any particular moment in life. Discovering and claiming our unique identity is a process of growth, change, renewal, and regeneration throughout our lifetime. As a specific marker, identity may seem tangible and fixed at any given point. Over the life span, however, identity is more fluid. . . . Identity formation is the result of a complex interplay among individual decisions and choices, particular life events, community recognition and expectations, and societal categorization, classification, and socialization. (1998, p. 51)

To claim or form an identity, let alone be open to changing it, one must be willing to take a stand for and against what constitutes the elements of that identity. I don't believe Cynthia had the capacity to do that at the time she gave birth to her children. Her decision to have children may have been made out of a sense of what was expected of her as much as her own desire. Children who are not allowed to grow, flourish, and develop a sense of identity enter into adulthood being nearly children themselves. They can have a very vague and shadowy sense of who they are or might be and require a great deal of time and effort to unveil a fuller sense of self. Cynthia exhibits in her narrative a frequent uncertainty and vagueness when recalling events that exemplify her generally obscured sense of self. Her alcohol and drug use further exacerbated this obfuscation.

Cynthia's relationship with her husband and his parents further suppressed her fragile sense of identity as a woman and mother. She reports that her husband William would call her "mommy," favor their son over their daughter, expect her to do the domestic and child-rearing chores, and make important decisions without consulting her. William's parents never figure prominently in her story, in terms of support, and her mention of them suggests that her worth to them was as the mother of their grandchildren. William also used drugs and did not offer any help with raising the children until she started attending NA meetings. His later recalcitrance regarding her visiting the children and getting information about their lives further diminished her self-esteem. According to Cynthia's reports, he used the children as pawns against her.

This being said, Cynthia had ambitions for her life that went beyond the repetitiousness and routine of childrearing. I use the term ambition here in the way that Shari Thurer uses it:

> We are the first generation of women among whom many dare to be ambitious. But there is no getting around the fact that ambition is not a maternal trait. Motherhood and ambition are still largely seen as opposing forces. More strongly expressed, a lack of ambition—or a professed lack of ambition, a sacrificial willingness to set personal ambition aside is still the virtuous proof of good mothering. For many women, perhaps most, motherhood versus personal ambition represents the heart of the feminine dilemma. . . . in performing nurturance, in becoming stay-at-home mothers (should we have the luxury of that option), we fear that we are turning into our own mothers, complete with their low status, self-sacrifices, and frustrations. (1998, p. 245)

The powerful stirrings of an evolving sexual identity further complicated an already daunting task of finding her true self. Understandably, it appeared to be much easier for her to contemplate exploring her lesbianism given the privacy she would have living apart from her children. She may also have felt that having children was incompatible with a lesbian identity, since much rhetoric during the women's movement in the United States in the 1960s and 1970s decried the oppressiveness of having children (Polatnick, 1997). Kath Weston further illuminates this conflict:

> Many lesbian parents described motherhood as a status that made their sexual identity invisible. In their experience, heterosexuals who saw a lesbian accompanied by a child generally assumed she was straight and perhaps married. Before the lesbian baby boom, gay activists often challenged the presupposition by calling attention to the numbers of lesbians and gay men with children from previous heterosexual involvements. This information often surprised heterosexual audiences, but they were able to reconcile it with essentialist notions of homosexuality by treating these offspring as the product of earlier, "mistaken" interpretations of an intrinsically nonprocreative lesbian or gay identity. If motherhood can render lesbian identity invisible, lesbian identity can also obscure parenthood. (1991, p. 168)

In addition to other cultural, emotional, and social imperatives, her upbringing as a Catholic played a powerful role in shaping her responses and behaviors. Religious doctrine teaches what is bad and good, what is sinful and virtuous. My experience both personally and in my therapy work with clients suggests that these teachings, especially when introduced from an early age, encourage certain responses and behaviors. Being raised Catholic myself, and subsequently rejecting the religion, I was taught from an early age that guilt, shame, and suffering are feelings to be constantly integrated into one's moral code. The same can be said of Cynthia's case.

Tearing down these individual responses can be difficult because the responses are deeply connected to religious teachings and other social imperatives. In exploring the "motherhood mystique," Denmark, Rabinowitz, and Sechzer write:

> The images that we cull from religion, myth, fairy tale, and the mainstream media are stunningly similar and idealized portraits of young, well-groomed, usually slim and conventionally beautiful women. They are virtually always heterosexual, married to the fathers of the children, White, and middle class. In personality and orientation to their children, they are usually gentle, patient, loving, devoted, and self-sacrificing. They are basically

asexual; in fact, they have few personal needs and desire of any kind and certainly no negative proclivities. (2000, p. 290)

Growing up, Cynthia learned that being a good mother meant staying with the children, being subservient to her husband, rejecting the "sin" of homosexuality, seeking forgiveness for her resentments toward her son and daughter, and staying in a situation longer than she wanted or was healthy for her.

Feeling guilt allows Cynthia to feel better about leaving the children; she feels she needs to be punished, and guilt is that punishment. Cynthia felt deeply rejected by Scott's bouts of anger and withdrawal, and this may have produced a kind of replaying of her feelings of being a bad child herself, thereby explaining to her young mind her father's abuse toward her. Cynthia's mother also encouraged guilt in her children, as she did not stand up to the father's abuse. By allowing the abuse, she reinforced the belief in her children that they were indeed deserving of this abuse.

This is an extremely complicated psychological knot to unravel, one that was experienced as emotional turmoil rather than a cognitive understanding for Cynthia. Cynthia finds it extremely difficult to come to terms with the fact that she was not a bad child or a bad mother for being unable to cope with the challenges of raising two young children and ultimately deciding to live apart from them. If she can fully understand the former, she will be able to better understand the latter. It is precisely because she learned to think of herself as a bad child that her pattern of thinking so easily constructs her as being the bad mother.

The myth of the good mother is a powerful one. The good mother (implicitly and explicitly advanced as white and middle class) stays at home with her children, takes delight in every stage of their development, and extracts a huge sense of accomplishment and satisfaction from fulfilling her primary role of nurturer and caretaker.

[Motherhood] myths include the seemingly natural and common-sense notions that only women can be loving and nurturing enough to raise a child; that men are vocationally superior to women; that good parenting requires that one parent, virtually always the woman, regularly subordinate personal goals to the children's and family's needs; that motherhood is uniquely joyous and fulfilling for women; that a good mother is invariably kind, unselfish, and loving; and that motherhood is the ultimate way for women to gain esteem and support as adults. (Denmark et al., 2000, p. 290)

To the extent that her children are happy, thriving, well-behaved, smart, and attractive, a mother is viewed as good. If a mother wants or needs to work outside the home, she can retain her label of good if she finds excellent day care for her child or hires a nanny or other kind of in-home child care. But even then, the good mother is expected to come home from work and cheerfully take over her evening and weekend task of delighting in her child. As Virginia Held (1984) writes:

> A mother is expected to give up whatever other work may interfere with her availability to care for her child and to take full care of the child—cheerfully and contentedly, to whatever extent, and as long as the child needs it. And if it is thought that the child will develop problems due to early separations from a parent, it is the mother who is thought responsible for preventing them. (p. 8)

The bad mother is the one who finds her children a drain, or is bored by the day-to-day grind of caregiving or wants more in her life than her role as mother. She is imagined as the mother who drinks too much, is too tired to read bedtime stories, goes out at night to attend her painting class leaving the children with a babysitter. The bad mother is imagined as the one who demands that the father take equal responsibility for child rearing—the mother who insists that her time is as valuable as his. The bad mother is, of course, the one who neglects or abuses a child in her care. The ultimate bad mother is the one who no longer wants to live with her children, who has just had enough and says no.

> Mothers who "lose their children"—who do not seek or obtain custody of their children in divorce proceedings, for example— are viewed as stunning failures, often stemming from a lack of understanding about how mothers become noncustodial and from the common belief that only mothers can be good parents. (Grief as cited in Denmark et al., 2000, p. 292)

The bad mother who is also a lesbian and, therefore, imagined to be an immoral and deviant woman, is the ultimate evil.

Although an unlimited supply of messages say a good mother is one who puts her children's needs before her own, Cynthia's story illustrates that a woman needs to take care of and heal herself to be able to have a positive relationship with her children. Mothers who stay in untenable situations risk doing irreparable harm to themselves and their children. By healing herself, Cynthia saved her relationship with her children. She also provides for them a model in which a mother's well-being and integrity is as important as the children's. This is a great gift for both of them.

Cynthia was valiant in seeking support through professional channels. However, she felt abandoned by two therapists: the first because of homophobia, and the second because of Cynthia's unwillingness to take antidepressants during her initial stages of drug abuse recovery. At a time when she most needed surrogate parenting from a therapist, she felt betrayed by them. This echoed her own childhood and the prevailing sense of her own worthlessness and not being good enough. Cynthia was on her own in her middle-class, white, isolated nuclear family with a husband and two children. She was expected to do it all (Kitzinger, 1980), so she turned to the only resources available to her: therapists, doctors, and support groups. Although the help Cynthia received when leaving the marriage was positive, her ambivalent feelings about being a mother were not adequately addressed.

With a more supportive kinship structure or already-in-place community ties, Cynthia may have been able to find the help she needed on a more or less informal basis. Extended families and community networks exist in some ethnic cultures. As Patricia Hill Collins writes:

> For women of color, the subjective experience of mothering/ motherhood is inextricably linked to the sociocultural concerns of racial ethnic communities—one does not exist without the other . . . [W]omen of color have performed motherwork that challenges social construction of work and family as separate spheres, of male and female gender roles as similarly dichotomized, and of the search for autonomy as the guiding human quest . . . This type of motherwork recognizes that individual survival, empowerment, and identity require group survival, empowerment, and identity. (1998, p. 233)

In her comparative analysis of how a Black women's group and a white women's group viewed motherhood, Polatnick notes that the Black women's group considered motherhood a source of power for women: "[T]hey defined the mother role more broadly; it encompassed caring for all the children of their community and fighting for a better future for the community" (1997, p. 389). She goes on to say that

> with educational and job opportunities extremely limited, teenage [Black] girls saw no future more appealing than motherhood. Having a baby was their main route to adult status . . . the emotional satisfaction of having a baby loomed large in this impoverished environment. Furthermore, [their] lives centered on kin and neighborhood networks in which mothers were the key figures. Being a mother was a major source of positive identity for these women. (1997, p. 393)

Cynthia's fear of losing all access to the children because of her sexual identity appears key to her decision to leave unchallenged the court's custody arrangement. She did not have great faith in her lawyer. Her internalized homophobia as well as the political realities of lesbian mothers receiving unjust and discriminatory treatment within the judicial system presented a set of obstacles too daunting to manage. Equally plausible is that Cynthia's need for the privacy and freedom to explore her lesbianism may have been limited if she had had more responsibility after the divorce for childrearing.

The list of challenging circumstances continues with the clinical depression diagnosis. Had this depression been discovered earlier in her life and proper medication prescribed, Cynthia's ability to take on the demands of mothering may have been significantly stronger. Today, Cynthia is a certified drug and alcohol abuse counselor, married to her female partner for three years, and enjoys what I observe as a healthy relationship with her two teenagers. Although she is now battling a new diagnosis of multiple sclerosis, she faces life's challenges head on. There is still work for her to do in understanding the larger mosaic of her life and the ways in which her circumstances and environment have produced the range of choices available to her. I have every confidence that the integration of her best emotional, spiritual, intellectual, and mothering selves are in her future.

Cynthia's story provides an opportunity to examine our preconceived ideas about the loaded concept of choice as it relates to mothering and motherwork. Cynthia had enormous obstacles to overcome, which were exacerbated by her unpreparedness to raise two children. She now lives apart from her children as a result of what seems like choice. Cynthia's story invites serious examination of the diversity among women, the social imperatives that impact differently on different women, and the limited range of viable options available to them as mothers. Her story entreats us, as counsellors, friends, and mothers, to imagine and support alternative ways of mothering that are healthy for women and their children.

REFERENCES

Collins, P.H. (1998). Shifting the center: Race, class, and feminist theorizing about motherhood. In L.J. Peach (Ed.), *Women in culture*. (pp. 231-244) Malden, MA: Blackwell.

Denmark, F., Rabinowitz, V., & Sechzer, J. (2000). *Engendering psychology: Bringing women into focus.* Needham Heights, MA: Allyn & Bacon.

Gil, E. (1988). *Treatment of adult survivors of childhood abuse.* Walnut Creek, CA: Launch Press.

Held, V. (1984). The obligations of mothers and fathers. In J. Trebilcot (Ed.), *Mothering: Essays in feminist theory* (pp. 7-20). Totowa, NJ: Rowman & Allanheld.

Herman, J.L. (1997). *Trauma and recovery,* Second edition. New York: Basic Books.

Kirk, G. & Okazawa-Rey, M. (1998). *Women's lives: Multicultural perspectives.* Mountain View, CA: Mayfield Publishing.

Kitzinger, S. (1980). *Women as mothers.* New York: Vintage Books.

Polatnick, M.R. (1997). Diversity in women's liberation ideology: How a black and a white group of the 1960s viewed motherhood. In R.D. Apple & J. Golden (Eds.), *Mothers and motherhood: Readings in American history* (pp. 389-416). Columbus: Ohio State University.

Thurer, S.L. (1998). Fall from grace: Twentieth century mom. In Lucinda Joy Peace (Ed.), *Women in culture* (pp. 244-255). Malden, MA: Blackwell Publishers.

Weston, K. (1991). *Families we choose: Lesbians, gays, kinship.* New York: Columbia.

Chapter 5

Sandy's Story: Re-Storying the Self

Lekkie Hopkins

> Multiple stories feed into any text; but, equally important, multiple selves feed into the writing or performance of a text, and multiple audiences find themselves connecting with the stories which are told. (Lincoln, 1997, p. 38)

As a feminist academic responsible for teaching feminist knowledges to (mostly) mature-aged undergraduate women, I am fascinated by the ways we come to know and by the changes that occur for us when we absorb new ways of seeing new knowledges. During the latter half of the 1990s, I worked closely with a group of students investigating the process that I have come to call "re-storying the self" in the light of current feminist understandings of the complex fluidity of subjectivity and power. My central participant in that research project was Sandy Newby.*

Sandy became a student at the university in her early forties. As a young woman, by her own account, she was silenced.

SANDY: My university education gave me new ways to read the events of my life. For a long time, for years and years before I went to uni, I actually used to feel I was outside my life looking in. For so long I couldn't get into it. But then at uni what I had been in the past didn't need to limit me anymore. What mattered now was the potential I had—to use my emotions as well as my intellect, to think creatively, to learn more, to open my eyes to what people had been thinking and doing for centuries and to what we might be able to think and do in the future. I felt loosened, freed up, so that the idealized me that I carried inside, the me who was possible and potential, was now within my sights. I could reach towards her and know she was possible.

---

*Pseudonyms have been used for all persons with the exception of Sandy Newby who chooses this forum to tell her story.

Sandy's story seemed simultaneously representative of the stories of many of her student colleagues and yet unique. Until she went to the university, she rarely felt that she was heard. Immediately on graduation, she became a trade union activist. She spoke in terms of voice and audience. I was intrigued to follow her re-storying processes more closely.

This chapter foregrounds a seminar presentation that Sandy gave as part of a unit called "Working with Women in Minority Groups." Students' seminar presentations in this unit occurred within a context of contemporary feminist investigations of ways to make spaces for (different) women from minority groups to speak. The lecture series occurred within the broader context of historical understandings of the development of feminist activism in Australia in the past three decades. The lectures challenged taken-for-granted notions of power being monolithic and immovable and embedded in institutional structures. They also challenged notions of personal identity being coherent, predetermined, and fixed.

In the lecture series I drew on the work of Australian scholars Jan Pettman (1992), Anna Yeatman (1995), Catherine Waldby (1995), and Ien Ang (1995), among others, to argue that such postparadigmatic understandings of power and subjectivity created the need for a new and different suite of collective practices from those used in the past. To make spaces for (different) women to speak, students needed to be able to recognize and respect difference, align momentarily and strategically over sameness, and learn consciously to read and shift power in interpersonal and group encounters. Such practices would be underpinned by consciously held feminist ethics.

"Sensitivity to difference may recognize the variety and specificity of women's experience, and the resulting groups may become smaller and more particular" (Pettman, 1992, p. 156).

In the lecture series, I argued, too, that the desire to create a positive, vibrant, energetic space from which every woman can speak of her difference has emerged as a significant dimension of the feminist project, particularly in the past decade, with its emphasis on differences among women and the politics of representation. Understanding this, I argue, is crucial for working across sites of difference, using reciprocity, empathy, and respect.

To begin grappling with these feminist notions of working across sites of difference, students were encouraged in their seminar presentations to draw on their own experiences of marginalization. Sandy's seminar presentation was about her experience of being cast as an unbecoming mother. It had a profound impact on her listeners, creating a moment that she and I have come to see as an epiphanous moment in her university life. What follows is Sandy's story as she presented it in class and our entwined understandings of her process of re-storying her self.

SANDY'S SEMINAR PRESENTATION

It was 1986. America's Cup fever was gripping Perth, and it seemed we were all caught up in the fervor that was the eighties. I had a "model" marriage—a devoted husband and two lovely daughters. I had a casual job to supplement the family income and my husband's career was on track with a recent promotion. We had built and moved into a new home in the suburbs in 1983. For all intents and purposes my life was set.

But I had a dark secret. A place within me where the inner struggle to survive was a daily familiarity. I had always been told I was headstrong and that my radical opinions were inappropriate, so I deduced that the difficulties I was experiencing were mine. So, never being one to take commitment lightly, I set about fulfilling the predetermined expectations that lay before me.

As described so exquisitely by Adrienne Rich (1979), I experienced both deep joy and indescribable agony as I tried to fulfill my mothering destiny. At every step I fell short of the "ideal mother" that existed inside my head. Guilt became the mother of my existence. My sense of isolation, both from myself and the experience I came to view as the real life that lay somewhere out there in the real world, created a spiral of confusion and anger. Depression became a constant companion and tears flowed endlessly.

No matter how marginalized any woman may seem to be, she is always, at the moment of articulation, at the center of her own story. Or as Susan Stanford Friedman argues, "To themselves, people made peripheral by the dominant society are not 'marginal,' 'other.' But to counter the narratives of their alterity produced by the dominant society, they must tell other stories that chart their exclusions, affirm their agency (however complicit and circumscribed) and continually (re)construct their identities" (1998, p. 230).

In 1986 I left my marriage. I left my children with my husband. Simone was six and Celeste was only two. As I remember it, my reasoning went something like this . . .

I have to have freedom or I will die . . . I am a bad person and a failed mother.

I don't know what lies ahead for me and I know I am unstable . . . the children need stability.

I am hurting my husband so much by leaving; I will destroy him if I take the children too . . .

My husband has a good income and will be able to support the children. I have no qualifications; I don't want my children to live in poverty . . .

I suffered an immediate loss of all my support networks—friends and family. I lost my identity. The housewife role had never felt comfortable, but it had been my source of status. In the years that followed, my search for identity and my emotional vulnerability led me into relationships and experiences which were, at times, devastating.

Having stepped out of my mold I found myself in quicksand. I had never lived away from my family, and my emotional survival skills were very limited. I lost my point of reference. Men saw me as single because my children didn't live with me. I saw myself as a person with irrevocable ties to my daughters. Other women were harsh judges. I gave up trying to explain or be truthful. Often, I chose not to let people know I had children, and yet they were and still are an enormous part of my life. I was always committed and available to my girls.

Initially, my husband felt that my sharing a rental house with other people added up to a bohemian lifestyle, which could not be tolerated. Although I was having constant contact visits with my daughters, I had to prove stability to him before we could come to an arrangement about weekend visits. This took about six months. Both of us were reluctant to use the legal system for our negotiations. My family rallied around him to support him through the crisis. My mother cooked for him and helped with the children. The realization that access to their grandchildren was no longer secure forced my parents to renegotiate their relationship with my husband.

I remember the night my grandfather on my father's side died. Unknowingly, I called my father for a chat, which at that time was not a common occurrence. My timing was impeccable. The rest of my family, including my husband and children, were gathered at his house because of the death. No one had called me. I had never felt like more of an outcast.

After the separation, I was consumed and disabled by the guilt I was feeling. I had left everything behind. When we finally did settle our property, I took the minimum amount possible so that Alex wouldn't have to sell the house and to ensure the family's stability. I tried to pursue joint custody but was advised by my lawyer that this was not an option (something I found out much later was not correct). So settlement included joint guardianship and sole custody to my husband.

Although I had always worked (casually or part-time after my children were born), without qualifications I was receiving wages at the lower end of the scale and my rental commitments were large. Other than the early days, I have rented accommodation that was suitable for my children to come and stay with me. This has been every weekend, some midweek, and some holidays since the early days of negotiating. The rent was often more than I could realistically afford but, for me, providing an appropriate environment for the girls was paramount. When I did secure a long-term position, I was employed as a functions and outdoor catering coordinator, which was very demanding of my time, including weekends. Trying to balance work with weekend child visits was a nightmare.

The unrelenting economic hardship I was suffering placed additional pressure on my somewhat shaky emotional health. The fear surrounding being the absent parent has created an instability which has been difficult to manage. The degree of suffering and long-term sadness I have felt culminated, as recently as last year, in treatment for post-traumatic stress syndrome.

In retrospect, I can see that I had to reconceptualize what my role was, who I was. In the time since I have been a noncustodial mother, I have learned many things–about myself, about the society in which I live, about how to be a mother when you are viewed as not being a mother. As I think back over the years, I can now identify my experiences as ones of redefinition

of my self concept

of myself in relation to my family and friends

of myself in relation to my husband

of myself in relation to my employers

of myself in relation to the state

of myself in relation to the ideology of motherhood.

Over the years I have found myself mediating family problems for my husband and daughters and dealing with emotional difficulties as they arose— from afar. I have had to maintain a degree of contact with my husband which allowed me to involve myself in family relationships but which somehow created some distance. This has been very difficult. In some ways, it has felt like the marriage has not ended. I have been trying to find a space for myself which allows me to express my individuality but which displays the level of commitment to my daughters that I feel. They have always known of my love for them and connection to them.

"First she dies. Then she loves. I am dead. There is an abyss. The leap. That Someone takes. Then, a gestation of self—in itself, atrocious. When the flesh tears, writhes, rips apart, decomposes, revives, recognises itself as a newly born woman, there is a suffering that no text is gentle or powerful enough to accompany with a song. Which is why, while she's dying—then being born—silence" (Cixous, 1991, p. 36).

Pain has been my constant companion, grief and loss my daily reality. Most of all has been the battle to allow me to be who I am and wanting people to see me as a person rather than categorizing me according to my actions and their perceptions of them. Underpinning all of my efforts had been an internal process of peacemaking and understanding. I have tried to rise above my culturally ascribed "proper" role and to express my individuality.

Always present, however, is the inner critic that quietly attacks. The part of me that struggles to come to terms with the actions of a mother who left her marriage. The part that seeks acceptance of myself, by myself. I have, at times, been my own harshest critic, and yet I know that my actions arose out of a desire to end the suffocation, to end what, for me, had become a nightmare. The cost, however, has been great.

In her analysis of this story from her own life, Sandy explored the limitations of pre-postmodernist feminist tendencies to generalize while theorizing women-as-a-category:

Without accommodating different speaking positions within its framework, feminism in the past has allowed generalized representations of women-as-a-category to permeate cultural consciousness. Thus, women's lives have been homogenized and many women's experiences and voices have been rendered invisible and inaudible, creating excluding practices rather than acting to include diversity. All women, therefore, are judged and are controlled and affected by implication (Pettman, 1992). Mothers-who-are-not-mothers become a threat to dominant voices, and to society as a whole, by stepping outside prescribed ideals.

She concluded her paper with a list of strategies that feminist workers could use to connect across difference with mothers-who-are-not-mothers.

FINDING A VOICE: GIVING LIFE TO HER STORY, AND A STORY TO HER LIFE

I know from my own response and from that of others that this has been a big moment for us all. It occurs to me now that I can read Sandy's narration of this episode in her life in terms of the conflicting discourses and desires it represents. Here is the quintessential feminist dilemma: the choices she makes are framed within a feminist ethics—responsibility to her (free) self is her primary achievement—and her struggles are to negotiate across the gaps between her self and other selves to persuade those others to read her as still responsible, loving, and caring, although she has shattered forever the myth of happy families and good mothers. In terms of a recent paper about desire by feminist scholars Susan Dormer and Bronwyn Davies (2001), Sandy's decision to leave her family acts on the desires for freedom that most women have and cuts across the equally powerful desire to be recognized as a good woman. The good woman is aligned with the unfree woman. Desires conflict. Goodness equates with entrappedness; freedom equates with badness.

"To find a voice. What does it mean? What does it mean when a woman finds her voice? And when she finds it, what then? . . . I mean she found a voice that narrates, orders, considers, reconsiders, backtracks, and gives life to a story, and a story to her life" (Modjeska, 1990, pp. 93-94).

The huge shift that Sandy makes, and that many in her audience may well have read as courageous in the extreme, is that she has been able to re-read, re-cognize, re-narrate her actions using a suite of understandings (feminist knowledges), which allow her to bring into being personally held feminist ethics underpinning her decision. She has found a voice. Drusilla Modjeska's (1990) notion that to find a voice means giving life to a story and story to a life resonates with those of my favorite theorists. In Irigaray's terms, "giving life to a story" suggests removing all boundaries, celestial and earthbound, and engaging with jouissance, with excess, with the chaos of the feminine imaginary to evoke the fluidity, multiplicity, and intertextuality of feminist knowledges; "giving story to a life" suggests an ongoing reflection on the art of writing a narrative, honoring both the temporal and the spatial to create the story in feminist ways that work out of the feminine imaginary, combining an aural economy with a scopic economy to bring the feminine subject into the symbolic. There is much movement here. This is not a static process.

Irigaray's quest for an alternative female symbolic calls into question every step of the process of becoming-subject, from the relation to the origins and consequently the maternal, to the transcendental, to one's relation to time and history; Irigaray's project consequently sexualizes in the feminine the very structures of subjectivity. An elemental sort of female cosmology pervades Irigaray's work: a firm, even shocking determination to return to the female imaginary the colours, the shapes, and the tempo of women's passions, her thoughts, as sexed female. A sensible transcendental foundation for a female process of becoming-subject (Braidotti, 1994, p. 112).

To make sense of how we might undertake a re-storying of the self, I link my understanding of Drusilla Modjeska's conception of the production of voice (that is, that voice is born of the movement implicit in giving life to a story and story to a life) with Elspeth Probyn's (1993) understanding that voice comes from the interstices of knowledge and experience. I link these understandings with Pam Morris's (1993) call for a theory of the subject that will allow for political agency and the production of voice, through a strategic process of self-narration that is historically, culturally, and sexually contingent. My intuition of the significance of the movement implicit in narrating the decentered, complex, and contradictory self and in connecting with others to become activist has led me to focus my attention on the hybridity of the space between sites of difference. This in turn has led me to the emphasis on reconceptualizations of space and time embedded in narrative scholar Susan Stanford Friedman's (1998) work on what she calls "the geographics of identity."

Out of such conceptual braiding has come an understanding of ways to build on the creative tension embedded in the simultaneous acknowledgment of difference and sameness, both interpersonally and collectively. Friedman's (1998) work provides a recent example of original thinking in this area. In reflecting on the doubled understanding of the term identity as being born of difference from unlike others, as well as from sameness (as in the term identical), Friedman brings together her own work on narrative with the work of such scholars as Trinh Minh-ha, Homi Bhabha, Gayatri Spivak, and Chandra Talpade Mohanty to use spatial and locational discourses to create what she calls a "geographics of identity": difference versus sameness; stasis versus travel; certainty versus interrogation; purity versus mixing: the geographics of identity moves between boundaries of difference and borderlands of liminality (Friedman, 1998). Such a discourse allows her to articulate "not the organic unfolding of identity through time, but rather the mapping of territories and boundaries, the dialectical terrains of inside/outside or centre/margin, the axial intersections of different positionalities, and the spaces of dynamic encounter" (1998, p. 19).

This kind of geographic discourse allows Friedman to read both interpersonal and collective engagements across sites of difference and sites of sameness. It often emphasizes not the ordered movement of linear growth but the lack of solid ground, the ceaseless change of fluidity, the nomadic wandering of transnational diaspora, the interactive syncretisms of the global ethnoscape. Although my work in this particular research process rarely crosses ethnic or national boundaries, I have adapted Friedman's geographic discourses to read moments of tension generated by the difference-sameness divide at various points throughout Sandy's journey toward feminist activism. Turning Friedman's work to my own ends, at the end of this chapter I undertake a mapping of the performances and negotiations that occur for Sandy in the hybridity of the space between a number of sites of difference.

In Sandy's seminar presentation, she reads and narrates her actions against the grain of all those discourses, which would position her as bad mother, abandoning mother, inadequate woman. She inhabits a space that says simply, My actions were informed by love and re-spect: love of the self ("I had to escape or I would die"); love of my daughters ("the children need stability"); respect for my husband ("I will destroy him if I take the children too"). At the same time, she re-mains her own harshest critic ("always present . . . is the inner critic, that quietly attacks").

The price she pays is high, as her story of the night of her grand-father's death reveals. The glimpses of detail from the daily life of the family that has closed ranks against her ("my mother cooked for him and helped with the children"; "I had to prove stability to my husband before we could come to an arrangement about weekend visits") serve to emphasize Sandy's marginalization and exclusion. However, in spite of the pain of such marginalization, she knows deeply that her decision has been responsible, ethical, and right. Her decision holds within it the glimpse of a future, which would have been impossible without her move.

My reading of the significance of this moment, in educational terms, is that it rests in the relationship between speaker and audi-ence. In this classroom, Sandy had a space in which she could power-fully speak the unspeakable, the abject. She could speak the story of the bad woman and not be rejected, but instead recognized as brave, and as offering truths for herself and for others. Her voice, as Probyn (1993) suggests it must, came directly from the interstices of her (feminist) knowledges and her experience. In addition, she writes against the grain of the kinds of feminist knowledges that celebrate motherhood as an inevitable source of power and satisfaction. It is not surprising that her audience was electrified.

As researcher/biographer, in an acknowledgment that truth or reality cannot be conveyed except in a way that simultaneously reveals their relativity and their relationship to the voice which speaks them (Thomson, 1994), I seek other responses to this moment of articulation in Sandy's life.

I talk to Lorna, media student par excellence. She is in her mid-twenties, young for this course. Sometimes she wears squashy velvet hats to class. Her whole demeanor embraces difference. She has a big personality. I know from observation that she and Sandy connected with each other quite strongly during this class, but I have not asked either of them how until now. Lorna's response, as it ought, takes me by surprise.

I really liked and respected her as a person, and when she stood up and said those things about her kids and what had happened in their lives, it really blew me away. It changed my relationship with my own father and mother completely. My father had abandoned me when I was four, and I never saw him again until I was nineteen. I'd always seen it as abandonment, and I had always felt it was about me, that I wasn't a good enough child, because if I was he would have struggled to be with me. But Sandy's story made me rethink my parents' stories. Suddenly I saw them as people who had been struggling with their own lives. And I remember we were all just about crying. Very special. I can't even remember my own assignment for that class, but I remember hers.

Lorna goes on:

My mum's not diagnosed but I'm sure she's manic-depressive. I mean she'd have great sunny days and we'd go and do all these things, and then she'd be drinking and down and trying to kill herself and stuff. In my autobiography I say I have healed the scars of my mother's disinterest. I call it disinterest; it's not abuse, or hatred, or whatever. It's just disinterest. Her happiness in her life did not include her children. Strange. And I think that's another way I connected to Sandy's story, because she so obviously felt grief about her motherhood and her situation, and I felt y'know some people do want kids to start with. Recently at the coexistence concert there was lots of talk about the Stolen Generation, and I said to my friends, I wish someone had stolen me from my parents! It's a difficult thing to say, but I would have loved to have been stolen.

Almost two years after Sandy's crucial seminar presentation, Sandy and I talk about that moment of articulation again.

SANDY: So yeah, there was . . . toward the end of my university studies there was a definite claiming . . . The claiming process was huge in that unit, where I gave the talk about my experience in your class, about, y'know, the noncustodial parenting aspect of my life, and going public with that, because that was part of a very dark secret I rarely ever told anybody because of the judgment that always followed. And that was really a moment of claiming of who I was, to myself, or who I had been, or even in terms that Drusilla Modjeska would use, claiming and telling that particular story of that part of my life—acknowledging that being a noncustodial parent was also part of who I was. It was really hard. Well, you were there. You could see it was really hard for me to do that. I can see now that I used university in a way that was challenging and meaningful and scary I guess in a lot of ways . . . It was interesting, the reaction of the class, because at that time I'd become fairly friendly with Verity who was in the class then, and she said to me afterward, "I just couldn't look at you, because I would have been sobbing so loudly it would have ruined everything," and um . . . who was the other young woman who was the filmmaker in that class? Fantastic personality.

LEKKIE: Oh! Lorna!

SANDY: Yes, Lorna. We'd been skirting around the fringes of each other, and in fact she's a very powerful woman, and in some of the groups we'd been in together we didn't actually agree at all on the . sort of positions that we'd have; and she came up to me afterwards, and she was . . . she was really blown away, and she said, "Oh I'm just, I just don't know what to say. It's amazing. I would never have guessed that this had been your experience, and y'know it's changing the way I think about my whole life already."

It is clear from these transcripts that Sandy herself reads this performance as a significant moment in her storying of her life. The metaphors she uses are of release, of floodgates opening:

SANDY: That was a huge day for me, because it really unlocked my heart that day. For some reason I took myself off to see *Priest*, the movie, that afternoon, on my own. It was a movie that I'd heard about, knew nothing about, but everyone said "You must see *Priest*." Well, by the time *Priest* was finished I was actually sobbing hysterically and couldn't stop, and actually I cried for about ten hours after that. I just, it was like the floodgates had opened, so I'd started some sort of release that had obviously needed to happen for a very, very long time.

It is clear, too, that the metaphors she uses here and elsewhere are implicitly about moving from darkness into light: she was no longer hiding; her dark secret was uncovered and out in the open; she could be an honest person (in the light) now.

SANDY: So the process of university is part of my healing, but also part of becoming an honest person, and not hiding. I still don't talk about that part of my life a lot, but I . . . I can say it in conversation now without feeling like a horrible person. And that seminar presentation, coming clean in that way, certainly had a huge part to play in that. But I was also able to go to the feminist theory in my essay that I wrote to support it. That gave me a position on it that I'd never had before, that said to me "Well this is how this happened to you." So there was an understanding there, that I didn't have before, and it was wonderful.

LEKKIE: Mm, mm. The most wonderful kind of experience of integration and flowering.

SANDY: Yes, it was. Yes, it was an amazing day, that. Scary stuff, though, but good stuff.

REFLECTIONS ON THE RE-STORYING PROCESS

What was it that was so significant about this seminar presentation for Sandy, in terms of her re-storying of herself to enable her emergence as a feminist activist able to understand the plays of power in working with and across difference to make changes?

The comments Sandy makes about her storying process draw me to reflect on Trinh's (1989) discussion of knowledge and consciousness and writing the self. Here Trinh draws on her experience of Eastern philosophies to argue that "thought is as much a product of the eye, the finger, and the foot as it is of the brain" (p. 28). She critiques Western self-satisfactions to argue that ego is an identification with the mind: "when ego develops, the head takes over and exerts a tyrannical control over the rest of the body" (p. 28). Trinh deftly eludes the Eastern/Western binary opposition then to offer a solution that once again takes us into the territory of reciprocity:

> If it is a question of fragmenting so as to decentralize instead of dividing so as to conquer, then what is needed is perhaps not a clean erasure but rather a constant displacement of the two-by-two system of division to which analytical thinking is often subjected. (1989, p. 39)

Trinh also refers to the procedures which, in Asia, postulate not one, not two, but three centers in the human being: the intellectual (the path, connected with reason), the emotional (the oth, connected with the heart), and the vital (the kath, located below the navel, which radiates life. It directs vital movement and allows one to relate to the world with instinctual immediacy). But as Trinh points out:

> [I]nstinct(ual) immediacy here is not opposed to reason, for it lies outside the classical realm of duality assigned to the sensible and the intelligible. So does certain women's womb writing, which neither separates the body from the mind nor sets the latter against the heart . . . but allows each part of the body to become infused with consciousness. (1989, p. 40)

Sandy's own comments on what happened for her on the day of her seminar presentation, and my subsequent reflections on that event, suggest that hers is an example of someone who is beginning to bring together Trinh's three centers in the human being: the intellectual, the emotional, and the vital. Sandy framed her presentation intellectually within a suite of feminist knowledges that allowed her and her audience to understand her actions as necessary and ethical in her own terms; she spoke with authenticity out of her own experience of pain and grief (the vital); and, in her own words, performing in this way "really unlocked my heart," so that after the presentation was over, "the floodgates opened and I cried and cried for about ten hours."

Such bodily responses can be seen to have profound impacts on how and what we come to know. As Elizabeth Grosz argues:

> Putting the body at the centre of our notion of subjectivity transforms the way we think about knowledge, about power, about

desire . . . and this entails the possibility of forming other kinds
of knowledge, other kinds of social interactions, other forms of
ethics, other systems of representation based on different interests, not only those of women, but those of cultural others . . .
whose bodies are inscribed in different forms and therefore
whose subjectivities and intellectual frameworks are different
(as cited in Somerville, 1999, p. 219).

Furthermore, in terms of Probyn's notion of "speaking with attitude," Sandy's performance here can be seen to have "put into motion
the doubledness of being and becoming" (Probyn, 1993, p. 163). In
her performance she can be seen to have looked back not to wallow in
her own misery but to read it anew. Her authentic immersion in her
own state of being, which allowed her to bring together Trinh's three
ontological centers, can be seen to have propelled her to the edges of
the known self, thrusting her into the doubledness of being and becoming of which Probyn speaks.

Finally, in terms of Drusilla Modjeska's (1990) account of finding
voice, Sandy can be seen to have given life to her story through con-
textualizing it within feminist knowledges and through acknowledging the complexity of tensions and storylines acting on her as the central character in the drama of her life: the good mother, the mother
who leaves to save herself; the good wife, the wife who feels trapped;
the lucky woman, the woman who is suffocating; the rebellious daughter, the daughter who seeks approval; the suffering woman, the woman
who is shriveling up inside. That she gave a story to this complex
background, which acknowledged her pain and vulnerability as well
as her strength and compassion, suggests to me that she was indeed
speaking out of the interstices of knowledge and experience, finding a
way to speak that somehow freed her from the constrictions and limitations of reading her life according to the old discourses that were so
successful in drowning her in her own guilt.

Here, then, is what we might call an epiphanous moment in
Sandy's university life.

And now, I turn to my own ends as a feminist pedagogue wanting
to make sense of the intricacies of negotiating the self. I draw on Susan Stanford Friedman's (1998) notion of the mapping of the performances and negotiations that occur in the hybridity of the space between a number of sites of difference. Sandy's articulation in her
seminar presentation of her experience of being a "mother-who-was-

not-a-mother" can be mapped as a moment of encounter between the (feminist) ethical transgressor and the (feminist) desiring audience. The space she inhabits is underpinned by feminist ethics. This suite of ethical discourses, though, runs counter to many mainstream discourses still informing the values and attitudes of many members of her audience. They are disarmed by the shock of this encounter with such a clear example of the disruptive implications of feminist knowledges (which they also endorse). She tells her story from the perspective of someone who has acted ethically, out of love and respect for self, children, husband. She tells her story to an audience whose capacity to imagine her pain and her experiences of marginalization provide the energetic support she craves. She becomes the speaker of the unspeakable. Her contradictory and extreme experiences of pain and marginalization and love make sense here in the context of feminist ethics. In drawing unwaveringly on her experience and on her knowledges, both new and old, she becomes for the first time able to articulate the enormity of her pain and the complexity of her reasoning. She moves from margin to center in her own storying of her life. She has spoken, and she has been heard. She knows the power of disruptive performance.

REFERENCES

Ang, I. (1995). I'm a feminist but . . . "Other" women and postnational feminism. In B. Caine & R. Pringle (Eds.), *Transitions: New Australian feminisms* (pp. 53-73). Sydney: Allen & Unwin.

Braidotti, R. (1994). Of bugs and women: Irigaray and Deleuze on the becoming-woman. In C. Burke, N. Schor, & M. Whitford (Eds.), *Engaging with Irigaray: Feminist philosophy and modern European thought* (pp. 111-137). New York: Columbia University Press.

Cixous, H. (1991). *Coming to writing*. In D. Jensen (Ed.) & D. Jenson (Trans.), *"Coming to writing" and other essays by Hélène Cixous* (pp. 1-59). Cambridge, MA: Harvard University Press.

Dormer, S. & Davies, B. (2001). Desire and the re-cognition of selves. *The Australian Psychologist, 36*(1), 1-6.

Friedman, S.S. (1998). *Mappings: Feminism and the cultural geographies of encounter*. Princeton, NJ: Princeton University Press.

Lincoln, Y.S. (1997). Self, subject, audience, text: Living at the edge, writing in the margins. In W.G. Tierney & Y.S. Lincoln (Eds.), *Representation and the text: Re-framing the narrative voice* (pp. 37-55). Albany, NY: SUNY Press.

Modjeska, D. (1990). *Poppy*. Ringwood, Victoria: McPhee Gribble.

Morris, P. (1993). *Literature and feminism*. Oxford: Blackwell.

Pettman, J. (1992). *Living in the margins*. Sydney: Allen and Unwin.

Probyn, E. (1993). *Sexing the self*. London and New York: Routledge.

Rich, A. (1979). *Of woman born: Motherhood as experience and institution*. London: Virago.

Somerville, M. (1999). *Body/landscape journals: A politics and practice of space*. North Melbourne: Spinifex Press.

Thompson, H. (1994). *Biofictions*. Townsville: Foundation for Australian Literary Studies.

Trinh, T.M. (1989). *Woman, native, other*. Bloomington and Indianapolis: Indiana University Press.

Waldby, C. (1995). Feminism and method. In B. Caine & R. Pringle (Eds.), *Transitions: New Australian feminisms* (pp. 15-28). Sydney: Allen & Unwin.

Yeatman, A. (1995). Interlocking oppressions. In B. Caine & R. Pringle (Eds.), *Transitions: New Australian feminisms* (pp. 42-57). Sydney: Allen & Unwin.

Gentle Even With Garbage

Si Transken

. . . And.

How is your son?

How is your son?

for 24 years a bland question endured
awkwardly
regarding the stranger who angled into my world
    after a New Year's Party
where i lost track.

arrived in the same month as my own birth.
left that day
on his own journey with strangers
who got stranger every year.
week end contacts
monthly if they allowed it.
his eyes were never entirely his father's.

And.

do people each week,
month,
year,
ask his biological father about the son,
the party,
where losses & tracks went?
that town scratched & skimmed every scrap from me

that could be taken
& another town,
job,
province,
opened possibilities
& my son said 'no' to stepping off the track
he found himself on.
relocation,
different connection,
how it might have been.
strangers estranged him from me
& his sense of humor which mirrored mine.

And.

i think a lot about garbage:
the kind we eat,
wear,
carry,
give away,
get thrown at us,
become.
my son collects the stuff for a city.
he's paid well,
is respected in his beliefs about jesus,
redemption,
loyalties,
consistencies.
silences.
a man making his world matter in his own ways.
aligned with aliens,
understandably
he won't speak to me
on Xmas day
or any other with that cadence similar to my own.

And.

biology's not destiny.
family's a contrived combination of chaos,
law,

biology,
a strangle of remembrances,
erasures,
a tangle of fibs,
funny stories,
lies,
pragmatics,
diplomacies,
accidental affinities,
habits,
hobbies.
mostly i chose to be unfamilied.
this cuts down on therapy,
pharmaceutical supports.
i've become garbage taken out.
last i heard he was still writing stories.

And.

i tire of teaching,
talking,

trembling about legacies
& lies.
wanting now to be in other fictions
and fabrications which don't gloom 5,000 years of tarnish.
doing our work in different geographies
under the stare of the same unconcerned sun
we get cash for collecting
& organizing garbage.
he freely signed up for extra English classes way back
     when he was a kid.

And.

his eyes were never precisely like any i'd seen before.

PART II:
PERSPECTIVES FROM THE OUTSIDE
LOOKING IN

Chapter 6

"Forsaking Their Children": Distance, Community, and Unbecoming Quaker Mothers, 1650-1700

Susanna Calkins

In 1662, Joan Brooksop left her children and husband in Berkshire, England, in order to venture across the Atlantic Ocean to the Massachusetts Bay Colony, disregarding the Puritan commonwealth's repressive legislation against her religious sect, the Society of Friends (or Quakers). Inspired by a prophetic missionary impulse to make the harsh and rigorous journey, Brooksop sought to warn the people and authorities of Boston that God's judgment was upon them and to persuade them to find the light of Christ within themselves. With this vision in mind, Brooksop traveled throughout the Caribbean and the colonies of North America for several years, suffering public whippings and stints in prison. In her later memoirs she recognized that her extensive travel caused a complete and undeniable rift between her family and herself. Paraphrasing Scripture, she reasoned that fulfilling God's will was right and good even though she had "forsaken all my relations, Husband, and children, and whatsoever was near and dear unto me; yea and my own Life too, for his own Names sake . . ." (Brooksop, 1662, p. 12).

Brooksop was one of many Quaker women in seventeenth-century England who left their children for extended periods of time, often journeying great distances across Europe, the Middle East, and North America, to fulfill their mission as the handmaidens of God. Fulfillment of this religious mission often had heavy, and perhaps unforeseen, costs. In addition to lengthy voyages away from their homes, many Quaker women were separated from their families by imprisonment, banishment, and community scorn. For example, Jane Christin and Alice Cord were separated from their children and husbands after being permanently banished to the Isle of Man for publicly preaching in 1668 (Penney, 1913). Alice Hayes was stigmatized and emotionally distanced from her family after an alleged altercation in which her father-in-law screamed, "Do not Thee and Thou me" (Hayes, 1765, p. 17). He cursed her and

> in a most despising manner said, a Quaker! Away with it; If you had been any Thing else; had you been a Baptist, and gone to hear them every day in the week, it had not been so bad as this. (Hayes, 1765, p. 17)

Similarly, Miles Halhead blamed his wife for their son's death, claiming that it was God's judgment for her rebellious nature (Barbour, 1986). Anne Camm, who traveled extensively across England and was frequently imprisoned for months and years at a time, would at her deathbed still call for her estranged son whom she had ceased mothering at a very early age (Trevett, 2000). Adding insult to injury, satirists of the day regaled their readers with raunchy accounts of "she-Friends [who] freely offered themselves with much cheerfulness to accompany the Brethren into any region whatsoever" (Anonymous, 1689).

Quaker women moved from a state of virtuous and legitimate motherhood to a delegitimated category of women who had left their children in what Gustafson (2000) calls an "unbecoming process." Yet, paradoxically, these female Friends reshaped the social prescriptions toward motherhood that underscored the expectations for women in the Early Modern era. In response to their own misgivings and the communal scorn they faced for abandoning their children, many Quaker women refashioned themselves as spiritual mothers who had been commanded by God to look after the needs of all Quakers, not just those of their own families. Through letters, personal testaments, and sermons, these "unbecoming mothers" detailed their own virtues and confirmed their value as prophets, teachers, and leaders. Even as female Friends ventured great distances from their children, many wrote extensive tracts that outlined their expectations for motherhood and proposed ethical guidelines for raising children. Instead of becoming "nonmothers," such strategies enabled Quaker women to reshape their understanding of motherhood and to reclaim legitimacy and virtue through their new and broader identities as spiritual and community mothers.

EARLY MODERN MOTHERHOOD

In Early Modern England, the idea prevailed that a disciplined family was at the heart of the social order. In the most simplistic sense, wives were expected to obey their husbands, servants their masters, and children their parents. In return for this obedience and fidelity, the head of the household, more a benevolent patriarch than a tyrant, was expected to perform his duties as husband, father, or master properly and to maintain the family livelihood (Amussen, 1988). Women, idealized as "chaste, silent, and obedient," were expected to maintain their homes in a godly manner and to oversee the spiritual and physical nourishment of their husbands and children (Hull, 1982, p. 1). Such ideas were derived from Scripture, disseminated in household manuals, and affirmed in children's catechisms (Charlton, 1999; Mendelson & Crawford, 1998).

In this period, children were viewed as the reward of God, and husbands and wives were expected to follow the biblical injunction to go forth and multiply. Clergymen urged women to avoid contraceptives and to shun abortion in expectation of God's mandate. Physicians, assuming that all men and women naturally desired children, wrote advice manuals for midwives (and expectant mothers) that endeavored to teach women how to protect their infants before and after birth (Charlton, 1999; Culpeper, 1653; Sermon, 1671). Women who were unable to conceive were regarded as tragic figures, as were women who gave birth to stillborn infants or children with deformities (sadly called "monsters" in Early Modern England). Women who used contraceptives or had abortions were almost as poorly regarded as women who committed infanticide or murdered their children.

A good mother prayed heartily and consulted astrological charts, such as John Pool's *County Astrology* (1650), even before conception to ensure the most auspicious period for pregnancy and birth. A good mother read the handbooks on pregnancy or, if she was illiterate, used the services of a highly knowledgeable midwife or an even more knowledgeable and learned physician. A good mother took care of her body during pregnancy, from conception through gestation, to birth and breastfeeding, through infancy and weaning her child from her breast (Charlton, 1999; Salmon, 1994). William Gouge, a prominent physician, declared that a mother's particular duty for her children began in the womb:

> A mother must then have a tender care over herself when she is with child for, the child being lodged in her and receiving nourishment from her (as plants from the earth), her wellbeing tendeth much to the good and safety of the child. (Gouge, 1622, p. 505)

Good mothers were not to get angry, dance, or lift heavy objects while pregnant. Nicholas Culpeper advised pregnant women to exercise in moderation, to get ample rest, to get proper nourishment in order to "recruit a tired brain," to maintain their health, to "comfort the limbs," to "quicken the spirits" and in general to "make the body, senses, and spirits strong." Such methods, Culpeper avowed, would certainly result in strong children (1653, pp. 115-117).

Women were not just charged to take care of themselves during pregnancy; physicians and ministers urged women to breastfeed their babies with the life-giving force of their own bodies. Religious writers likened the nursing mother to God; the act of breastfeeding, in the religious imagery of the times, was like being cuddled in God's bosom (Salmon, 1994). Thus, women who breastfed their children were respected, while those who opted not to breastfeed, especially those who were physically capable, were criticized for shunning their children. As William Gouge heartily admonished: "Be not so unnatural as to thrust away your own children" (1622, pp. 18-19).

Injunctions for "good" motherhood did not seem to change as children grew older. Sermons and advice manuals were directed at parents of older children, advocating the parents' need for personal observation and close physical proximity to their children. Parents, especially mothers, were expected to watch over their children's health and to ensure their mental and spiritual well-being (Charlton, 1999; Salmon, 1994). Richard Baxter, a nonconformist, advised parents to be careful in the way they raised their children. He admonished them to raise their children on a "temperate and healthful diet" and to keep them busy in order to avoid idleness of mind and body (Baxter, 1624, p. 5). Mothers were to be diligent, keeping their children from pursuing vices ("gaming for money, from cards, dice and stage plays, play books and love books and foolish wanton tales and ballads") and from acting with "untoward familiarity with tempting persons of another sex" (Baxter, 1624, p. 5). In his ethical guidelines for child raising, Edward Lawrence warned that parents had to be present to teach their children Holy Scripture, and "to encourage them in the good, and discourage them in evil" (1681, p. 71). Although most advice manuals agreed that physical correction was to be used as the last recourse, "it is better thy child be whipt than damned" (Lawrence, 1681, p. 71).

Quaker literature concerning the education and discipline of children did not vary to any great extent from the prescriptive norm in mid to late seventeenth-century England. George Fox, the founder of Quakerism, had followed the seventeenth century expectation that children be raised in the fear of God, calling for Friends to "Train up all your children in the fear of God in his new covenant of light and grace, that they may know Christ" (Homan, 1939, pp. 8, 54). William Penn advised parents to love their children wisely, to explain "the folly of their faults," and to use the rod sparingly and judiciously (Penn, 1771, p. 1). "Never strike in passion," he warned, "and suit the correction to the age as well as the fault" (Penn, 1771, p. 1). In a letter to his children from prison, Isaac Pennington (1667) reminds them to recognize, respect, and obey the voice of God; to be virtuous in their deeds and thoughts; and to obey their parents. Similarly, Gertrude Niesen directed parents to guide and control their children, keep them in good conscience and fearful of God, and use "the Rod of a gentle chastisement" as necessary (Niesen, 1677, pp. 3-5).

THE PARADOX OF QUAKER MOTHERHOOD

Quaker women who left their children to go on spiritual journeys violated expectations for good mothers commonly held in mid to late seventeenth-century England. First, Quaker mothers were not purified ritualistically after childbirth, nor did they have their babies baptized, two expectations of good motherhood held by the Anglican Church (Trevett, 1991). Second, Quaker mothers often ignored the expectations for good motherhood established by the medical community. It is unlikely that the sight of pregnant women ("women in travail") or new mothers withstanding long bouts in prisons or traveling long distances by foot or horseback would be considered favorably by physicians or midwives.

Most physicians and midwives would have frowned upon Quaker women such as Esther Biddle who gave birth to at least one of her four children while in prison; Katharine Jackson who saw two of her newborn children die during her imprisonment at Warwick jail; and Anne Whitehead, later a confirmed "mother in Israel," who was imprisoned in Ilchester "away from her husband, and four small children, and one tender child she carried in her arms" (as cited in Hobby, 1992, pp. 37-38). Their religious beliefs, combined with the hardships they endured on behalf of their faith, set most Quaker mothers apart from the idealized mother envisioned by contemporary English society.

Even more significant, Quaker women who traveled great distances from their children occupied an ambivalent position within their own community of Friends. A dichotomy exists in Quaker literature and experience about the roles and expectations for women, especially in regard to motherhood. On one hand, there was a ready acknowledgment that Quaker women, as spiritual equals and the handmaidens of God, were as likely as their male counterparts to be called by God to preach in public, to rail against church and state authorities, to suffer punishment and imprisonment, and to travel great distances (Mack, 1992; Trevett, 1991, 2000). Such women were generally admired and held in great respect. As such, female Friends were not overtly criticized by Quaker leadership for leaving their children, husbands, and homes, for it was understood that this choice was not their own but rather the dictates of their "inner Spirit." It should be noted, too, that members of the Society of Friends referred to themselves as the "Children of Light," a telling name which suggests that, like true children, their innocence and virtue would be protected in a corrupt world by God, the father of all. Although this did not, by any stretch, negate the importance of the biological mother, the assumption was that God watched over and protected all of his faithful followers even in the absence of a parent.

On the other hand, there was an assumption of good motherhood in Quakerism that was at odds with the activities pursued by handmaidens of God and female prophets. As in the prescriptive literature concerning childhood, the Quaker mother was implicitly expected to be present and attentive to the spiritual and physical needs of her children. Quaker mothers, like other English mothers, were expected to teach their children the proper ideas about God, the right way to behave, and the right way to carry themselves with one another and in society. Most Quakers' letters and testimonies exhorted parents, especially mothers, to be watchful and attentive toward their children. They were expected to keep their children in sight to ensure virtuous behavior and to admonish and even discipline them physically as required. A good mother would not let her child be vain, foolish, idle, or led into temptation (Ingle, 1991; Mack, 1992; Trevett, 1991, 2000). The virtues extolled in this literature implicitly assume that a good mother is physically present, corrective, and watchful of her child.

The need for the physical, caregiving, nurturing presence of the Quaker mother was never so pronounced, nor so poignant, as when her child lay dying. In 1677, Joan Whitrowe collected and edited a number of testimonies that described the final moments of her fifteen-year-old daughter Susannah's life. The cause of Susannah's death was not made clear, but the authors of several of the testimonies hint that the girl had been involved in an illicit romance that was frowned upon by her parents and the local Quaker community and had been vain and frivolous in her actions. Implicitly, her illness was a sign of God's displeasure. For six days, her mother and various Quaker friends maintained an anxious vigil at her bedside, praying and recording Susannah's final excited visions and earnest penitent speeches to God, compiled later by her mother in *The Work of God in a Dying Maid* (1677). The girl chastised herself for her vanity, berated herself for bringing shame to her family, and lamented her alleged statements criticizing the local Quaker women's meeting. Joan Whitrowe withstood it all with a mother's "quiet and patient bearing" (Whitrowe, 1677, p. 3).

In many ways, Susannah's death and her mother's reaction to it symbolized the paragon of Quaker virtue and piety held for Quaker children and their mothers. In her death, Susannah offered an ideal modeled by a Quaker child that showed the simplicity and strength of true faith. In her dying epiphany, Susannah realized that her transgression was not simply defiance of her mother and the secretive relations with her unnamed suitor, but for her failure to uphold the Quaker ideal. She duly repented her wayward actions and lack of faith and, in an even more dramatic denouement, gave her body and soul to Christ in her deathbed conversion.

Even more significant, the narratives describing Susannah's death seem designed to underscore her mother's own piety, virtue, faithfulness, and devotion. In comparison, Susannah's father played only a small role in the tragedy, relegated only to a nebulous figure of questionable paternal authority. Repeatedly, Susannah affirmed Joan Whitrowe as a good mother and as a good Quaker. Allegedly, she avowed that "I have heard them say, that my Mother is so grounded in her Religion, that it is impossible ever to turn her. My mother is grounded indeed, she is established upon the Rock that shall never be moved . . . her name is written in heaven" (Whitrowe, 1677, p. 31). Most important, Joan proved herself a devoted caretaker and spiritual nurturer for her child, markedly never stirring from her daughter's bedside.

With the image of the attentive, nurturing mother so prominent in contemporary writings and in the words of their own sect, it is not surprising that many Quaker women who left their children to follow the will of God were clearly uneasy or anxious over their actions. Many of their children were, after all, either in an important moment in their early physical development or, perhaps more significantly, in an even more critical stage of their Quaker consciousness. Quaker scholar Christine Trevett (1991, 2000) suggests that many wives and husbands stayed apart from each other in a deliberate attempt to minimize pregnancy, as the presence of young children impeded women's abilities to carry out their mission for God. Most Quaker mothers denied, with heartfelt conviction, that this was their decision or choice, avowing instead that the impetus to leave their families came from a command from God that could not be ignored.

In 1670, Elizabeth Stirredge was called by God to leave her young children and make a dangerous hundred-mile trek to London (a very great distance in the Early Modern era). She was compelled to plead with King Charles II that he end the rigorous persecution of Quakers and reestablish their religious freedom. Allegedly stunned by the divine command, Stirredge later wrote:

> I did not think that the Lord would make of such a contemptible Instrument as I, to leave my habitation, and tender children to go to King Charles which was an Hundred miles from my habitation, and with such a plain testimony as the Lord did require of me, which made me go bowed down many months. (1810, p. 37)

In 1658, Sarah Chevers and Katharine Evans left their children and husbands in England, having been called by God to travel to Alexandria in Egypt. At the whim of the ship captain, the pair was forced instead to disembark in Malta, a stronghold for the papal Inquisition. Undaunted by the change in their plans, the pair began to distribute Quaker tracts and pamphlets, a provocative gesture that resulted in their imprisonment for the next four years. In addition to their most famous account of their captivity, *This is a Short Relation of the Some of the Cruel Suffering (for the Truth's Sake) of Katharine Evans and Sarah Chevers, In the Inquisition in the Isle of Malta* (1661), the pair also wrote several letters to their children and husbands still living in England. Evans declared that she prayed for her children every day, hoping that they would keep their faith in God, "keep a diligent watch over every thought and action," and avoid "the snares and baits of Satan," despite the prolonged absence of their mother (1661, p. 53).

Sarah Chevers offered similar sentiments to her children, urging them to remain steadfast in their faith, but closed her letter very differently. She was, quite likely, acutely aware of the contemporary attitude that a good mother remained in close physical proximity of her children. Chevers first reminded her children that she had been justified by God when she left (and essentially abandoned) her young family. She assured them that she had not left the family for her own pleasure and that her impetus had been solely at the command of God. Expressing the harsh reality she encountered in Malta, she wrote:

> I cannot by Pen or Paper set forth the large love of God in fulfilling his gracious promises borne in the wilderness, being put in prison for God's truth, there to remain all days of my life, being searched, tried, examined upon pain of death among the Enemies of God and his Truth; standing in Jeopardy for my life. (1661, p. 56)

She then explained, as many Quaker women living apart from their children did, that she believed that separation between them was only physical. Spiritually, she considered them to be joined in God's love and through mutual faith they would "have community [with one another] in spirit" (1661, p. 56). By keeping and sharing the same faith, she explained, they would remain in spiritual communion despite being physically separated by an immense geographical distance and despite her death, which she believed imminent. By asserting her position as one of God's chosen agents, she could ignore contemporary opinion that she be physically close to her children and allay any of her own misgivings. As such, she could still retain the spiritual and didactic authority expected of the seventeenth-century English mother.

Perhaps the anxiety over a Quaker mother's separation from her children can best be seen in Joan Vokins, a Berkshire Quaker, who felt her inner spirit beckon her to North America in 1680. Vokins, a self-described "sick and lame woman" resisted "the dictates of [God's] spirit" so that she would not have to undertake the arduous journey to New England and leave her children and husband. From the outset of *God's Mighty Power Magnified* (1691), a lengthy tract narrating her hazardous journey through the Caribbean and the colonies of North America, Vokins asserted her authority and position as a handmaiden of God, albeit one on the brink of death. She never desired to travel or to write for her own sake. On the contrary, she claimed modestly that she would rather stay in the comfort of her own home, surrounded by her children and husband, and rest her wearied, sickly body. She could not, however, refuse the command of God.

> I could take no comfort in Husband or Children, house, or land, or any visibles, for want of the marriage with the lamb of God ... If I had disobeyed the Lord, to please them, I might have provoked him to have withholden his mercies from us all, and to bring his judgments upon us. (1691, p. 18)

Finally, in a letter to Friends in New York, Vokins defended her actions:

> The feeling of [God's] sweet refreshing life that he communicates to my soul, is a hundred-fold better than husband and children, or any other outward mercies that he hath made me partaker of, though very near and dear unto me. (1691, p. 66)

THE PARADOX RESOLVED: QUAKER WOMAN AS COMMUNAL MOTHER

The paradox of the Quaker woman as a handmaiden of God who traveled great distances, and the idealized mother who was expected to keep a close vigil over the actions and faith of her children, was partially reconciled when the unbecoming mother took on a new identity, becoming a spiritual mother of the community. Since the movement began in the mid-seventeenth century, there had been "Mothers in Israel." Women such as Margaret Fell, Joan Vokins, and Anne Whitehead offered solace, comfort, religious training, and physical and spiritual nourishment to fellow Friends (Barbour, 1986). Through their writings, travels, and spiritual activities, such women presented themselves as the keepers of faith, guardians of Quaker virtue, and spiritual mothers.

The early Quaker preacher Edward Burroughs called Margaret Fell, "oh thou daughter of God, and mother in Israel, and nourisher of our father's babes and children" (as cited in Gardiner, 1993, p. 219). A letter from Margaret Fawcett to Margaret Fell in 1677 salutes Fell: "thou hath been as a mother to many children, and I with many more have received strength and nourishment from thee" (Webb, 1865, pp. 298-299). Rebecca Travers, herself referred to as a "great mother," warmly told Fell, "I know thou hast the compassions of a mother" (Travers, 1688). Theophila Townsend, a lifelong companion of Vokins, recalled her friend as

> a nursing mother over the young convinced; and in her own fam-
> ily, great was her care and endeavours for her husband children,
> that they might partake with her of the everlasting comfort. Her
> care was great for her children; that they might come to a sense ·
> of Truth. (Vokins, 1691, p. 7)

To other Quakers, Vokins showed the same spiritual guidance and comfort, "ready to hold forth a hand to the weak, to help them on in the way of peace, and to watch over them for good, and encourage them in well-doing" (1691, p. 8). In a similar eulogistic testimony, Anne-Mary Freeman wrote of Anne Whitehead, "when I was but a child she took me into her care and tenderly educated, and helped me many years and I can truly say I honoured as my Mother" (Freeman, 1688, pp. 16-17). Clearly, "Mothers in Israel" were viewed by others and by themselves as beacons of faith and a source of comfort and unity within the Society of Friends.

Although Quaker literature also presumed the existence of a watchful father, it was far more common and accepted that most male Friends would be separated, whether voluntarily or not, from their families for great lengths of time. Quaker women had long learned to make do without their husbands by running their businesses, maintaining their farms and stores, and looking after the welfare of their children. Quaker women, informally at first and in organized networks later, had helped one another financially, materially, and spiritually when their husbands were away preaching, imprisoned, incapacitated, or dead (Mack, 1992; Trevett, 1991, 2000). Thus, the absence of fathers and husbands, although a source of concern, had long been assuaged by the activities of Quaker women. The absence of mothers, however, sharpened the void and intensified the need for parental controls. As a result, discipline and correction increasingly came under the direction of spiritual and community mothers—many of whom had left their children themselves—who led the local Quaker communities.

Female Friends, having fashioned new identities for themselves individually as community mothers, began to orchestrate a larger, more systematic realization of the enhanced position of the Quaker mother with the creation of Women's Meetings on both sides of the Atlantic. In 1674, female Friends in London, led by Ann Whitehead, carefully composed an epistle that specified to all Friends in outlying regions in England, across North America, in the other far-flung regions to which Quakers had journeyed, the written expectations for Quaker women. These expectations included visiting the sick and prisoners, relieving the poor, making provisions for the needy and those unable to work, and caring for widows and the elderly. Women were entrusted with ensuring the education and spiritual welfare of fatherless children and poor orphans. They were to stop "tattlers and false reports, and all such things as tend to division amongst us" in a concerted effort to maintain a needed unity among the women and the larger Quaker community (Whitehead & Elson, 1680, p. 1).

Moreover, the spiritual mothers of the community were imbued with the ability to teach and stand as models for the younger women. Such older "women in the trust" were expected to train the younger in that "which is good, sober and discreet, chaste and virtuous" so that they would love and obey their husbands and children, teach their own children to fear God, and to otherwise live in a decorous manner (Whitehead & Elson, 1680, p. 1). Special monthly and quarterly Women's Meetings were intended to ensure that each woman met regularly in her faith community, and that she and her children were perpetually "refreshed" in their faith (Ross, 1938, p. 40).

Through pamphlets and tracts, eulogies and testimonies, and letters intended for specific family and friends and larger, more public audiences, the virtue of the Quaker community mother and her value as a teacher and leader were repeatedly affirmed. Texts, epistles, travel narratives, and other written experiences of the spiritual mothers circulated throughout the Friends' communities on both sides of the Atlantic. Many were published, adding to the authority, legitimacy, and credibility of their words. In this newly self-fashioned identity, Quaker women gave themselves the authority to educate and discipline the sons and daughters of the Friend's community when the biological mothers were absent. Although the spiritual mothers never supplanted the biological mothers, the stature and authority they created for themselves within the Quaker community was great.

Margaret Fell Fox, the "Mother of Quakerism" herself, asserted the importance of the spiritual mother's duty from God: "My dear lambs though a woman may forget the sucking child of her womb, yet cannot [God] forget such" (Gardiner, 1993, p. 219). Essentially, they looked after one another's children and expected that others would do the same. Indeed, as Vokins wrote to her sister and brother-in-law, "Dear Anne Lawrence's children be in my mind as well as my own: I hope you will look after them in my absence that we may have comfort of their growth in truth" (Vokins, 1691, p. 55).

In effect, spiritual mothers—many of whom had once traveled great distances away from their own children—taught biological mothers how to raise their children in accordance with Quaker ideals. Women's Meetings on both sides of the Atlantic repeatedly admonished women to "train up your children in the blessed truth and fear of the Lord" and to "keep the yoke upon that nature that is proud, stubborn, or disobedient to parents, break that will in them betimes which comes from the evil one, and bend them while they are young, lest when they grow up you cannot" (Waite, 1688, pp. 16-17).

In letters to her family and the Women's Meeting in London, Vokins even urged Friends to take note of a practice she observed among members of the Quaker community in Barbados. Calling it a "good precedent concerning children," she described how children accompanied their parents to the Meeting where they "wait upon the Lord and are instructed" in the ways of the Quakers. They learned

Fox's catechism from their parents at home and were expected to re-
cite what they learned at the weekly Meeting under the guidance of
the community leaders (Vokins, 1691, p. 75). Lest anyone doubt the
power of the catechism within the children, Vokins explained that
"many of them was tendered and let tears when [she] was at their
Meeting" (1691, p. 75). The letters and epistles from the spiritual
mothers were meant to reassure themselves and one another. Simply
put, if a Quaker woman were compelled by God to travel to distant
lands, she should rest easy knowing that other Quaker mothers would
be attending to her children's spiritual and physical needs.

There is, however, a distinct silence in these tracts about how absentee Quaker mothers actually provided for the children they left behind, or if they made any plans at all. Although many tracts and travel
accounts suggest that the mothers left home spontaneously in response to the call from God, unless they traveled only on foot, they
likely had some time to prepare their families for their absence while
waiting to book passage on a ship. Some Quaker children, following
the practice of the times (Sommerville, 1992), may have been placed
as domestic workers or apprentices in the homes of Friends entrusted
to maintain their spiritual and physical well-being (Trevett, 2000).
Others may simply have been left under the care of their fathers. Joan
Vokins worried that her husband could not be entrusted to raise their
children properly in her absence. In a letter sent from Rhode Island,
Vokins urged her husband:

> to have an Eye over our dear Children, that they lose not the
> sense of Truth, which my Soul hath so deeply travailed for,
> when I was with them; for it is my fear, now I am from them, that
> if thou do not supply my place in my absence, that the Spirit of
> this World will prevail, and hinder the Work of the Lord in their
> Hearts, and in thine too, and that will be to all our Sorrow. (1691,
> p. 52)

Similarly, the responses of Quaker children toward their absentee
mothers are difficult to establish. Perhaps as their mothers desired,
the children understood that their mothers were answering a greater
call than their own cries. In a 1686 letter, Joan Vokins enjoined her
children to

remember how I have bred you up and consider what manner of persons you ought to be, now that you are come to years to understanding, that you may not grieve the spirit of the Lord, nor me, nor any of His dear children that you may be good examples to others. (1691, p. 104)

Perhaps some children of Quakers did not come to terms with the loss of one or both parents to the faith. This may explain why Anne Camm shamefully referred to her prodigal son who had apparently run off when he was young (Trevett, 2000). To an even greater extreme, Margaret Fell's son George, the only one of her children to eschew Quakerism, even tried to have his mother imprisoned in the 1670s (Trevett, 2000).

Evidence from the perspective of Quaker children toward their parents is scarce, however, and interpretation of children's activities and attitudes by Quaker writers should be subject to scrutiny. By and large, children did not write letters or personal memoirs themselves, and adults alluded to only the general physical and spiritual well-being of the children in their care. Similarly, in the ongoing debate of prescription versus practice, it is difficult to assess whether the pervasiveness of parental warnings to negligent children had any basis in reality. We cannot know, for example, whether the warnings against vice and sin directed to children of absentee mothers were designed to stop a rampant willfulness and lack of respect for Quaker ideals that actually existed, or whether the warnings simply reflected an idealized relationship between a pious mother and a virtuous child.

CONCLUSION

In many ways, Quaker women from seventeenth-century England challenged contemporary attitudes about motherhood and female propriety. Even in the process of "unbecoming" mothers, traveling great distances from their homes and leaving their children for great lengths of time, many of these absentee mothers began to redefine what it meant to be a mother (Gustafson, 2000). Many began to refashion themselves with new identities as communal mothers who looked after the spiritual welfare of all Friends, not simply members of their own families. In 1688, the Women's Meeting of York warned women to keep a virtuous life, "especially you are drawn forth to bear public testimony for the Lord and his blessed truth, keep you to the watch" (Waite, 1688, p. 18). In its most extreme, by the end of the seventeenth century, the Women's Meeting in Lancaster, England, had even begun visiting Quaker families at home to ensure that the children were being educated and disciplined properly. If parents were found lacking in their child-raising abilities, the members of the Women's Meeting gave themselves the authority to remove the children from the home and place them with other families (Mack, 1992).

Over the years, as scholars discussed the activities of the first generations of Quakers, female Friends who had traveled and left their children became incorporated into the Quaker historiographical canon. Their bravery, determination, and commitment to the Quaker cause were persistent themes in early Quaker writing, from Joseph Besse's (1753) hagiographical *Abstract of the Sufferings of the People called Quakers* to W. Beck and T. F. Ball's (1869) *London Friends' Meetings*. By 1925, Quaker historian Mary Agnes Best described Katharine Evans and Sarah Chevers, the women who traveled to Malta, as "a pair of respectable wives and mothers" who had been divinely commanded to spread the true light of Christ. Best wrote: "As mothers of young families, Katharine and Sarah did not rush toward the fires of martyrdom with undue haste. Freely and boldly they proclaimed their beliefs and insisted on their right to hold them" (1925, p. 117, 122).

Joan Brooksop and numerous other Quaker women may have forsaken their children in the fulfillment of God's command, but their very absence ushered in a new position of authority, propriety, and respect for Quaker women in the seventeenth and eighteenth centuries. These spiritual mothers taught, disciplined, and nourished the members of the Quaker community as their own children. Their motherhood became a cherished aspect of their religious struggles, and it mattered less that they lived portions of their lives geographically separated from their children. Thus, in becoming spiritual mothers to the Quaker community, these women challenged the contemporary image of the good mother by living apart from their biological children. At the same time, their admonitions concerning motherhood found in archival records reveal some of the historical roots of contemporary imaginings of the good and present mother.

REFERENCES

Amussen, S.D. (1988). *An ordered society: Family and village in England, 1560-1725.* Oxford, New York: Basil Blackwell.

Anonymous. (1689). *The Quakers art of courtship or, the yea-and-nay academy of complements.* London.

Barbour, H. (1986). Quaker prophetesses and mothers in Israel. In J.W. Frost & J.M. Moore (Eds.), *Seeking the light: Essays in Quaker history* (pp. 41-60). Wallingford and Haverford, PA: Pendle Hill Publications and Friends Historical Association.

Baxter, R. (1624). *The poor man's family book.* London.

Beck, W. & Ball, T.F. (1869). *London Friends' meetings.* London: F. B. Kitto.

Besse, J. (1753). *A collection of the sufferings of the people called Quakers for the testimony of a good conscience, from 1650-1689.* London.

Best, M.A. (1925). *Rebel saints.* New York: Harcourt, Brace and Co.

Brooksop, J. (1662). *An invitation of love unto the seed of God.* London.

Charlton, K. (1999). *Women, religion and education in Early Modern England.* New York: Routledge.

Chevers, S. (1661). To her husband and children. In S. Chevers & K. Evans, *A short relation of some of the cruel sufferings (for the truth's sake) of Katharine Evans and Sarah Chevers, in the Inquisition in the Isle of Malta* (pp. 56-57). London.

Culpeper, N. (1653). *A directory for midwives or, a guide for women.* London.

Evans, K. (1661). To her husband and children. In S. Chevers & K. Evans, *A short relation of some of the cruel sufferings (for the truth's sake) of Katharine Evans and Sarah Chevers, in the Inquisition in the Isle of Malta* (pp. 53-55). London.

Freeman, A. (1688). In A. Steevens (Ed.), *Piety promoted by faithfulness, manifested by several testimonies concerning that true servant of God Ann Whitehead* (pp. 16-17). London.

Gardiner, J.K. (1993). Rendering individualism: Margaret Fell Fox and Quaker rhetoric. In J.R. Brink (Ed.), *Privileging gender in Early Modern England* (pp. 205 224). Kirksville, MO: Sixteenth-Century Journal Publishers.

Gouge, W. (1622). *Of domesticall duties.* London.

Gustafson, D. (2000). Unbecoming behaviour: One woman's story of becoming a non-custodial mother. *Journal of the Association for Research on Mothering, 3*(1), 203-212.

Hayes, A. (1765). *A legacy; or widow's mite* (3rd ed.). London.

Hobby, E. (1992). *Virtue of necessity: English women's writing 1649-88.* Ann Arbor: University of Michigan.

Homan, W.J. (1939). *Children and Quakerism: A study of the place of children in the theory and practice of the Society of Friends.* Berkeley, CA: Gillick Press.

Hull, S.W. (1982). *Chaste, silent, and obedient: English books for women, 1475-1640.* San Marino, CA: Huntington Library.

Ingle, H.L. (1991). A Quaker woman on women's roles: Mary Penington to friends, 1678. *Signs, 16,* 587-596.

Lawrence, E. (1681). *Parents groans over their wicked children.* London.

Mack, P. (1992). *Visionary women: Ecstatic prophecy in seventeenth-century England.* Berkeley: University of California Press.

Mendelson, S. & Crawford, P. (1998). *Women in Early Modern England 1550-1720.* Oxford: Clarendon.

Niesen, G. (1677). *An epistle to be communicated to friends.* Colchester.

Penn, W. (1771). Advice to children. In J. Fothergill (Ed.), *Select works of William Penn* (pp. 75-76). London.

Penney, N. (Ed.). (1913). *Extracts of state papers relating to Friends, 1654 to 1672.* London.

Pennington, I. (1667, rpt. 1847). Letters of early Friends. *Friends Library, 11,* 446.

Pool, J. (1650). *County astrology.* London.

Ross, I. (1938). Lancashire women's quarterly meetings minute book. *Journal of the Friends' Historical Society, 35,* 40-43.

Salmon, M. (1994). The cultural significance of breastfeeding and infant care in Early Modern England and America. *Journal of Social History, 28,* 247-269.

Sermon, W. (1671). *The ladies companion, or the English midwife.* London.

Sommerville, C.J. (1992). *The discovery of childhood in Puritan England.* Athens and London: University of Georgia.

Stirredge, E. (1810). *Strength in weakness manifest: In the life, various trials, an Christian testimony of that faithful and servant of the Lord* (2nd ed.). London.

Travers, R. (1688). A testimony concerning our antient and dear friend Ann Whitehead. In Steevens, A. (Ed.), *Piety promoted by faithfulness, manifested by several testimonies concerning that true servant of God Ann Whitehead* (pp. 24-25). London.

Trevett, C. (1991). *Women and Quakerism in the seventeenth century.* York: Ebor Press and Williams Sessions.

Trevett, C. (2000). *Quaker women prophets in England and Wales 1650-1700.* Lampeter, Wales: Edwin Mellen Press.

Vokins, J. (1691). *God's mighty power magnified.* London.

Waite, M. (1688). *Epistle from the women yearly meeting at York.* York.

Webb, M. (1865). *The fells of Swarthmoor Hall.* London: Alfred W. Bennet.

Whitehead, A. & Elson, M. (1680). *An epistle for true love, unity and order in the church of Christ.* London.

Whitrowe, J. (1677). *The work of God in a dying maid: Being a short account of the dealings of the Lord with one Susannah Whitrowe.* London.

Chapter 7

Unnatural Mothers:
Lone Mothers and the Practice
of Child Rescue, 1901-1930

Robert Adamoski

At the present time we have about 170 in the Home, and many of them are very young babies who have been deserted by their unnatural mothers . . .[1]

Across Canada, and in much of the Western world, social programs that defined the latter half of the twentieth century and much of what it meant to be a citizen have come under sustained attack. On the brink of their demise, a strong body of gender-sensitive analyses of welfare programs emerged, focusing on the specific forms of governance that these programs expressed, and their role in the creation of self-regulating, gendered, racialized, and classed citizens. This chapter examines some of the earliest policies and practices of the emerging Canadian welfare state and discerns important tendencies evident in efforts to constitute women as appropriately gendered citizens. These tendencies have reemerged in a starkly neoliberal form in recent policies directed toward lone mothers and their children (see, for example, Mink, 2001).

The following discussion focuses on the experiences of lone mothers in British Columbia who sought assistance from the Vancouver

I would like to thank the staff at the City of Vancouver Archives and, particularly, Head Archivist Sue Baptie, for their assistance with this research. Robert Menzies and Dorothy E. Chunn have supported this work with characteristic generosity and offered keen and constructive criticism; I thank them, and Diana Gustafson, for their contributions.

Children's Aid Society (VCAS) during the first three decades of the twentieth century. Correspondence and other data drawn from the case files of families who came into contact with the Society allow unique historical insight into how gender and race shaped the options available to lone mothers seeking alternate forms of care for their children.

The Society's policies and practices toward lone mothers highlight the gendered bases by which fathers and mothers were able to argue for standing as citizens in their contact with this emergent form of governance. I have shown elsewhere that lone fathers who approached the VCAS tended to be regarded primarily as legal citizens with guardianship rights typically respected by state agencies, provided they met their financial obligations (Adamoski, 1995). In contrast, women's relationships to their children are typically regarded as natural or innate rather than legal. Although fathers were, on occasion, chastised for attempting to foist their children upon public agencies, women who approached the Society for assistance in caring for their children were typically regarded as not only irresponsible but also unnatural.

In examining the Society's responses to the problem of lone motherhood, I also describe and analyze the Society's position among the myriad strategies by which women sought to meet their own needs and the needs of their children. The landscape of options was dotted with well-established charitable institutions and, during the latter years examined in this study, with emerging commercial maternity homes. The public nature of children's aid societies cast their relationship to families in a unique form. The characteristics that, according to the Society's spokesmen, distinguished it from charitable orphanages and commercial infants homes included a recourse to law, a concern to cultivate the province's Anglo-Saxon, Protestant citizenry, and a professed concern to arrest the further development of a criminal, pauperized class.

By understanding the fundamentally gendered character of child rescue practices during the period when citizenship was little more than a rhetorical construct for most women, we are better prepared to understand the gendered nature of the citizenship that evolved in later political contexts, including the maternal feminism that led to women's enfranchisement (Koven & Michel, 1993). Kealey has described maternal feminism as the conviction that woman's special role as mother gives her the duty and the right to participate in the public sphere. It is not her position as wife which qualifies her for the task of reform, but the special nurturing qualities which are common to all women, married or not. In some senses maternal feminism de-emphasizes or subordinates personal autonomy in favour of a (relatively) wider social role. (1979, pp. 7-8)

As this chapter illustrates, one enduring characteristic of citizenship in Western democracies is the importance of women's maternal and conjugal obligations in buttressing their political and social claims. As noted by Orloff, the bases on which women have been permitted to advance claims as citizens are most starkly evident in the different responses to the social problems presented by families

headed by a male breadwinner with an economically dependent wife (and children), and families maintained by women who are not in the paid labour force, or work on its fringes, who must make claims based on their status as mothers. (1993, p. 315)

The data examined here emerge from a larger study examining the policies and practices of the VCAS and a sample of 303 children from 154 families involved with the Society between 1901 and 1930. Drawing upon case files, correspondence, VCAS Annual Reports, Adoption Committee reports, and other organizational documents, the larger study traces the experiences of each family from their first Society contact until the discharge of each child. The limitations of case files as a historical source are widely recognized and have been carefully considered here. Nonetheless, there is wide consensus that these sources also allow unique insight into the experiences of individuals seldom recorded elsewhere. In the present instance, the files compiled prior to 1927 appear less filtered by standardized, bureaucratic, and professional convention. Most contain extensive correspondence between siblings, children, parents, Society officials, and foster parents. This chapter benefits greatly from these direct accounts.

Drawing data primarily from VCAS case files generally provides limited insight into the private options available to lone mothers raising children in this period. Nonetheless, exceptional cases document the censure that some women faced within their own families. One such case involved a family that operated a large, well-regarded dairy farm on Vancouver Island. They were, by all accounts, respected and financially stable. Excerpts from the running record provide the following clinical account:

> In the summer of 1925, . . . Mrs. Irvine [of the Nanaimo Children's Aid Society] visited the home . . . [and] found mother and R., aged 2 1/2 in a room in an attic living under most unsanitary conditions—faeces on the floor—no mattress on the bed, paper hanging in strips from the walls. . . . It is understood that R. had never been downstairs . . . [M]ost of the children are illegitimate as father deserted several years ago. . . . [Uncle Willis] states the whole trouble was the mother's illegitimate children. Her family do not feel they should be responsible for them.[2]

Five of the woman's children were committed to wardship and spent varying periods of time in the care of the VCAS. The family fought vigorously to have the two oldest boys returned to work on the farm in 1929, but when contacted about the possibility of taking "R.," the child whose infancy is described earlier, they were "sorry to say there isn't much doing in Nanaimo."

By comparison, of course, many of the mothers raising children apart from their biological or birth fathers were much more successful in their attempts to arrange for themselves and their children. In September 1924, R. Grayston—then superintendent and secretary of the Society—received a letter from A. M. Stephens, a long-time child rescue advocate. The letter outlined the concerns of Mr. J. M. Gilroy regarding the circumstances of his children, who were in the care of his estranged wife.

> I know that you have the power to . . . take these children into your custody, after investigation . . . Mr. Gilroy is able and willing to pay for the children's board and lodging etc. . . . These children . . . (aged 6 and 8) . . . are at present in the care of their mother, . . . who is not living with her husband but with a questionable character. This man, together with the mother of the children are engaged in running a "place" or "blind pig." The little children . . . are in this "place" exposed to the vileness and criminal influences of the surroundings. . . . They are neglected

if ever children were. . . . Every day that the children are left there is a serious matter affecting their future as citizens.[3]

In Stephens's eyes, women in the position of Mrs. Gilroy could not provide the moral and economic resources that her fledgling citizens required. Although his information was limited to that provided by the children's father, Stephens evidently found it credible, having little difficulty imagining that neglect of her children would flow inevitably from Mrs. Gilroy's lifestyle. Grayston visited the family shortly thereafter and recorded his findings.

> [The next morning] . . . I visited the home . . . and found the children with an Italian . . . apparently acting toward the children as father and mother, Mrs. Gilroy standing at the stove cooking something for a meal. . . . So far as the children are concerned they are well-fed and well clothed and during the day they are cared for by a young girl of 16 years of age . . . who lives on the opposite side of this Street. This girl stated that Mrs. Gilroy returns to the home generally about 1 A.M. and sleeps on the premises with herself and the children. . . . The influence exercised on these children must be very poor and the evidently close connection between the Italian and Mrs. Gilroy, which is undoubtedly of an illegitimate nature, must eventually tend to lead the children the wrong way. I propose to ask that these children be taken from both their parents as being unfitted to have control or direction of their lives.[4]

The majority of the lone mothers whose experiences are documented in the files of the VCAS occupied the continuum between the cases just described. Women, such as Mrs. Gilroy, who were able to construct systems of support usually avoided contact with men such as Grayston. Similarly, although cases of total ostracization appear, there is typically little definitive information about the circumstances of the parent(s) preserved on file. Instead, the portraits of families appearing within the Society's files were most often lone mothers who had long struggled to maintain their children with sporadic or nonexistent contributions from the children's fathers.

The construct of lone parenthood reflects and reinforces broader gendered practices. Elements of this phenomenon can be examined by deconstructing the lens through which officials of the VCAS (and others) viewed the social problems presented by lone mothers and their responses to those problems. In the sample, the largest percentage of lone mothers were characterized by the Society as being either parents of "illegitimate" children (30 percent of lone-mother families) or victims of "desertion" (28 percent). In comparison, none of the lone fathers in the sample had their children designated "illegitimate," while 21 percent were deemed to have been "deserted."

As they appear in the files of the VCAS, illegitimacy and desertion are fundamentally gendered, reflecting assumptions about naturalized gender relations and family structures, and utilized in fundamentally different ways by men and women within that context. Illegitimacy, as it was understood and wielded by officials of the VCAS, was intimately connected to the patriarchal, nuclear family structure, and reinforced by the historical ascendance of legal over social relationships. The concept continues to function as a historical foundation of the privilege attaching to male-headed families within the welfare state and the male archetype that continues to inform both legal personhood and nationalist citizenship. It should be regarded as integral to the gendered and racialized lens through which the families studied here were regarded.

Desertion and illegitimacy cases were similar in that they overwhelmingly involved mothers who had been denied the practical, emotional, and financial support of the children's father. They faced the mutually contradictory demands of "restoring the revenue deficit engendered by the absence of a man while still ensuring that domestic labour and childcare were performed" (Bradbury, 1993, p. 196).

Women who were successful in replacing the economic contributions of their husbands faced a more stringent test in the form of the moral requirements of motherhood. To men such as Stephens and Grayston, each element of the "web of means" (Bradbury, 1993, p. 196) that allowed Mrs. Gilroy's family to survive economically appeared to threaten the children's morality—the greatest threat being her extralegal relationship. Likewise, although all women faced with raising children alone in early twentieth-century British Columbia suffered from the contradiction between material survival and the stringencies of motherhood, women whose children were regarded as illegitimate were subject to the greatest challenges.

These so-called illegitimate children who were eventually committed to the VCAS were, in the majority of cases (60 percent of families), in the care of lone mothers at the time of first contact. In only two cases did lone fathers have custody of their children. The concern over illegitimacy as a drain on public resources was regularly expressed in the Society's organizational minutes and other published material. In the Society's Annual Reports for 1911 are the first explicit references to the perceived problem of illegitimate children.

> Your [Adoption] Committee has dealt with . . . numerous applications made to receive the offspring of misguided and unfortunate girls. Several girls have come to the city from various parts of Canada and some from the Old Land with a view to hide their shame and have made application. . . . Your Committee is of the opinion that the Society was not established for the purposes referred to in the previous paragraph.[5]

Again, in 1912:

> Applications are now being made to make children over to the Society and too often the request is made to cover up the crime of bringing a child into the world without a name and permit the mother and alleged father to pass through the world as being without a stain upon their character. Many of the little mites referred to were in a condition verging on to death.[6]

The imagery here reveals the stark effects of gender in the Society's policies toward lone parents. Paternity is presented as a legal status with criminal repercussions for the nameless child and an implied standard of due process to protect the rights of the "alleged father." The vulnerability of birth mothers seeking to avoid "their shame" lurks in contrast.

Similar themes emerge in a revealing piece of correspondence with the local press corps, wherein Charles ("C. J.") South—secretary, superintendent, and chief agent of the Vancouver Children's Aid Society for most of the period between 1901 and 1923—conveyed the circumstances surrounding the abandonment of a child whom he assumed was illegitimate. The child, being about two months of age, was found on the front lawn of a prominent family in 1913. South wrote of his "regret that the newspapers got hold of the transaction," saying, "I had requested them not mention this matter, for it is just an advertisement in my opinion, for women to leave their babies when they are not under observation."[7]

Here the "alleged father" disappears entirely from South's visualization of the problem of supervising mothers who allegedly awaited the opportunity to abandon "their babies." Given the hostile environment facing unwed mothers during this period, it is not surprising to find a number of poignant cases involving women pushed to desperation by the birth or pending birth of a child born outside of marriage. In many cases, information on file is limited to terse commentary by officials, not unlike the previous descriptions offered by South and the Adoption Committee. In other instances, case files allow for a more complete contextualization of the material and emotional circumstances in which these women found themselves.

In some instances, the correspondence and reports contained in these files beg for a degree of informed conjecture. One such case occurred in September 1913 when Officer Lowry of the Vancouver City Police brought an infant before Police Magistrate H. C. Shaw. The child had been found, apparently abandoned, in a boarding room in the city. The room was empty with the exception of a short, handwritten letter, unsealed and without an address. The letter and the court transcript (including Officer Lowry's testimony) offer the only available information concerning the child's identity and parentage.

> I answered call . . . where we found a baby girl about two weeks old. Mrs. Belleville of that address informed us that about 1 P.M. today a woman called there with this baby and asked for a room for one night which she got. She seemed to be very weak and sick. She said she had just come from the General Hospital. She then went to the room and wrote a letter . . . after which she went out leaving the baby on the bed. A short time after this some one phoned Mrs. Belleville enquiring about the child. This party said they were speaking from St. Mary's Hospital and that the mother of the child had fallen off a car and broken her back. Mrs. Belleville phoned all the City Hospitals, also St. Mary's Hospital New Westminster but could not find any trace of her. . . . We took the baby to the Salvation Army Home.[8]

Despite further exhaustive searches of Vancouver and New Westminster, authorities were unable to locate the mother, or find record of her hospitalization for either the birth or the alleged accident. The only information concerning the child's background came from the letter found with the child.

> Dear Sister—Just a few lines to let you know I'm still alive hope your the same but Gee I feel sick and weak. I just come out of the hospital today and I shouldn't of. I'm not fit to do anything. . . . My insides seems as if it was all on fire. There is something not right but the Baby is a darling . . . a little girl if its father was only alive to see her wouldn't he be proud. But still its all for the best. He's dead 8 months tomorrow. It seems strange for me to have a baby and him gone so long . . . I don't know anybody here in Vancouver and its very hard for me but strangers are very very good to me and everybody thinks baby is a dear . . . I have to get envelopes also before I can post this but there is a drug store right close and baby is real good hardly ever crys only when she's hungry. . . . With fondest love to all, Your loving sister Anna.[9]

Although officials of the VCAS did not explicitly categorize this child as illegitimate, the circumstances seem to suggest the desperation and inventiveness of individuals left only with undesirable choices. Such dynamics were further evidenced in the cases of desertion found in the files of the VCAS.

The case of the Chime family is typical of those in which mothers apparently deserted their children. In July 1909, the Chief Constable at Fernie, B.C., contacted C. J. South to ask for assistance in dealing with the family of John Chime, as they were in destitute circumstances. "It appears," the constable reported, "that [Chime] refuses to support his wife and family." The constable added that Mrs. Chime was "very anxious that two of the [three] children should go to the Children's Home."

Like many of the families examined in this study, the Chimes came to the attention of the VCAS primarily due to their desperate financial circumstances. In some cases, these families were deemed sufficiently deserving that South would consider boarding the children, and intervening personally in an attempt to convince the fathers involved to shoulder their responsibilities.

For Mr. Chime, and many other fathers, the policies of South and the VCAS had a distinctively less tolerant tone. South's primary concern in this instance revolved around methods by which Mr. Chime could be legally compelled to support his family. Refusing, in this case, to consider boarding the Chime children, South proposed that the primary response ought to be a legal one. Discussing the case with the provincial secretary, South fumed, "[i]f this man will not work and provide for his family then in my opinion he ought to go to jail and be made to work. I have advised the Police to this effect." The intersection of these gender and class-based policies typically had profound effects upon the decisions that faced women such as Mrs. Chime. Almost one month after first being apprised of the family's plight, South was informed by the constable that

> Mrs. Chime [had] left her husband and her whereabouts is unknown, leaving him with three children. The father . . . has made arrangements for the adoption of [the two youngest children, including a four-month-old infant] and there is a probability that [the oldest boy] being taken care of by some family.[10]

Instances such as these reveal the complexities that characterized desertion. Unable to obtain support from the police, the VCAS, or the provincial secretary, Mrs. Chime apparently pursued an option that promised some benefit for both herself and her children. A similar case reflects some of the dynamics evident in cases in which the VCAS agreed to become involved in an ongoing familial dispute.

In November 1911, Mr. Fritz approached the Children's Home and made arrangements to board his three children, aged nine, seven, and three years. After several months of unrest, his wife had fled the family home, initially taking the children. Unable to find adequate housing and without any real prospect of supporting the children, she had returned them to her husband, who had refused to allow her into the family home.

Just before Christmas 1911, Mrs. Fritz returned to the family's home and the children were returned. However, by February 1912, the children were once more on the Society's doorstep. This time, Mrs. Fritz had approached the Society asking that they again be boarded. In support of her application, she brought a letter from Reverend R. M. Thompson outlining the case.

> Mrs. Fritz . . . has asked me to do what I could toward the replacing of her children in the Home. According to her statement, she had them taken out before, because she could not endure being

separated from them, and because she hoped that the conditions in her home might improve. She is now quite hopeless and says that the children are not provided for in the matter of clothes and food, and she would rather suffer the separation than see them suffer want. . . . Personally I do not know her husband but it seems from what she says that there has been trouble between them frequently, owing to his gambling and non-support, and attitude toward religion . . .[11]

Although the children had been boarded at the Home only weeks prior, Mrs. Fritz's request to place her children in the Home was dismissed for lack of consent from the children's father. Discussions continued for several months, ending with a note indicating that Mrs. Fritz had again left her husband with the children, hoping to force him to place and financially support them.

Whatever the difficulties in distinguishing between desertion, mutually desired separation, and forced expulsion, we must conclude that it offered perils to women that did not confront lone fathers. In addition to the challenges that lack of access to a family wage presented for lone mothers, they found themselves subject to policies and practices that demanded a standard of conduct and range of responsibilities much broader and more nebulous than those demanded of fathers.

The case histories cited thus far reveal, in their actual practices and in the vocabularies with which they were reflexively linked, a naturalized vision of maternal obligations. Lone mothers were regarded as owing a natural or innate duty to their children, which was not mitigated by the desertion of their husbands or by their own poverty. The inability to meet this standard of naturalized motherhood rendered many of these mothers "unfit." Lone fathers were, of course, also subject to an evaluation of their worthiness to receive aid from the VCAS. In particular, the ability of the father to meet the financial obligations of boarding his children, attributed race and ethnicity, and any indication of leftist political leanings were carefully scrutinized. Nonetheless, lone mothers unquestionably faced a much more demanding standard in their quest for aid.

The consequences of the naturalized responsibilities of motherhood for lone mothers deserted by their husbands were significant. Lone women whose children were placed in the Home were more likely to have them apprehended than were men in similar circumstances. Furthermore, lone mothers who approached the VCAS seeking to board their children were most often denied this option. Sometimes the reason given was overcrowding, but this was often a blatant deceit. Although overcrowding was a chronic problem confronting the Children's Home, the boarding of children remained a common practice throughout the first three decades of the Society's existence. The preferential position of lone fathers as wage earners in British Columbia's economic structure was a key factor in their relative success in boarding their children. The following case, however, reveals that the gender structures that shaped the Society's policies toward boarders were not always reducible to simple economics.

In October 1913, Reverend C. Ladner of Kamloops wrote to the VCAS requesting aid for a woman who had apparently been successful in supporting herself and her three children for some years and wished assistance in boarding her children with the Society.

> A poor woman of this City has requested me to write you and ask if you could assist her in getting her two children into the Home. . . . Her husband went insane about 15 months ago—is now at Westminster—and there is no hope of his regaining his reason. She is left without means to support herself and children. She is now waiting on table in the best restaurant in the City, and out of her monthly income, could and would assist in meeting the keep of the children in the Home. . . . The case is a most distressing one. Will you please do all in your power to help her place her children in the Home.[12]

South's reply is representative of many similar cases encountered in this study. Despite her apparently exemplary character references and stable (if inadequate) source of income, the woman was denied aid.

> Regarding this poor woman you speak of: I am in great difficulty, for we absolutely are so crowded that I do not think at the present moment it would be possible to find room in the Home for even these two little ones. . . . In fact I would not like anyone to make us a present of a cat just now, for I don't know where we could put her.[13]

Lone mothers such as these, who were unable, by virtue of poverty, to provide an adequate home environment, were typically regarded by the officials of the VCAS as being unable to parent. In many of these cases, women who approached the VCAS requesting assistance in boarding their children were not merely denied service but were pressured to "voluntarily" cede guardianship.

In August 1914, South received correspondence from an Anglican minister in Nanaimo who detailed the circumstances of Mrs. Anheuser. She was held in some regard in her community for her efforts to provide for her three young children after the desertion of her husband some years earlier. Unfortunately, her health failed and the Reverend wrote to South asking for his aid in temporarily boarding the two youngest children while the oldest nursed Mrs. Anheuser back to health. South's reply blatantly repudiated the established practice of boarding at the Children's Home.

> I cannot take these, or any other children in the Home as boarders, as we have no room for boarders. If it is absolutely necessary that the children be committed to the Children's Aid Society as wards, some provision might be made . . .[14]

South proceeded to outline the implications of wardship, primarily the termination of Mrs. Anheuser's legal guardianship.

Mrs. Anheuser considered this change in guardianship to be her only available option and consented to making her second daughter Doris and youngest child Barbara wards of the society. For six months, she regularly wrote to the children and sent them gifts of clothing, shoes, and toys. Eventually, however, South wrote to advise Mrs. Anheuser that Barbara had been adopted and could no longer receive her letters. In a letter to South, Mrs. Anheuser responded this way:

> I would like to say that I was greatly upset to hear of my baby being adopted so soon. I suppose she will be dead as far as I am concerned. I expect it is the attitude of the association to keep their mothers in complete ignorance of their abode after adoption. I wish it would be a little more sympathetic. I would like you to know that I am not always going to be a helpless beggar. . . . I hope to be in a position to take Doris before very long. Do

you think there is a chance of my being able to see Barbara once in a while? . . . Thanking you for your past favours, etc. . . .[15]

In light of Mrs. Anheuser's account of the events that led eventually to the loss of her daughter, it is interesting to note the version of events that South gave to the family who adopted Barbara. South portrays Barbara's mother not as a member of a criminal class but as a noble (if tragic) figure.

I regret that I was unable to be with you the day you went out to the Home, but you have selected an exceedingly fine little girl. . . . The reason why Barbara and Doris came to the Home was through the death of their father, the Mother was absolutely destitute, and after considering for some time and trying to support her children, she found that it was absolutely useless to go on.[16]

Although she apparently never again saw her youngest child, Mrs. Anheuser was granted the opportunity to visit her older daughter Doris later in 1915. She wrote to South requesting the visit so that she might "reconcile [herself] to the hand of Fate." South's reply offers some insight into his understanding of the circumstances that resulted in the permanent separation of Mrs. Anheuser (a woman whose resignation he apparently regarded as appropriate) and her children. His reliance on a providential explanation is much more consistent with the fictional account offered Barbara's adoptive parents than it is with Mrs. Anheuser's own experience. Although South does not directly attribute blame to Mrs. Anheuser for the collapse of her family, he does little to acknowledge the role of her husband in the family's plight.

Of course when you come over if you will come to my office at the Dawson Block, corner of Main and Hastings Sts. I will be glad to give you an Order to go out and see Doris. . . . I got a letter two or three days ago about Barbara. She is very happy and contented, and they are very proud of her, as, under their tuition, she is fitting herself to occupy the position they intend their daughter to in the future. . . . Don't talk about the "hand of Fate." There is no such thing as Fate. All things that happen that we are not responsible for are permitted by One wiser than ourselves.[17]

South's decision to permit Mrs. Anheuser to visit Doris at the Children's Home, along with his accounts of the circumstances leading to the committal of the children, all illustrate his basic approval of Mrs. Anheuser as a conscientious woman who fulfilled the basic requirements of motherhood. The family lacked only a wage-earning father to meet the basic standard that infused the policies of the Society. However, even in cases such as these, South's actions reflected the prevailing attitude among both charitable agencies and courts of the day. These agencies generally appeared much more willing to sever the naturalized relationship between mother and child than they were to terminate the legal status of father.

As I examine elsewhere, legislation establishing Children's Aid Societies in North America involved the introduction of an alternative to the contractual indentures that had governed private transfers of guardianship and had supported some of the practices found in orphanages (Adamoski, 2002). This novel alternative created a form of public guardianship, which had the characteristics of being judicially imposed and ostensibly final.

Rather than invoking the more readily modified contractual agreements that applied to boarders, child rescuers relied on the strategy of terminating parental guardianship in favor of public guardianship. On occasion, this worked in favor of lone mothers who could no longer provide for their children. In May 1921, South received a letter from a woman who identified herself as Mrs. Thomasson, a widow living in the interior who wished to board her children at the Children's Home.

> Being a widow and labouring under great difficulties through the loss of my husband who was drowned 2 years ago, and, having two little children left on my hands I now feel that it would be to the best interest of the children and myself also to have them placed in a home, where they will be cared for properly. . . . Will you kindly send me full particulars as to what it will cost me to place my children in your home and conditions of payment. I could pay a small sum monthly if that would be convenient to you.[18]

South replied as he did to many such applications by lone mothers. Without inquiring into the circumstances or ever meeting Mrs. Thomasson and her children, he instructed her this way:

> When children are made over to the Society, the Mother loses the control of them. We are so crowded that we cannot take children in as boarders; they have to be made over to the Society absolutely, and then we have the right to adopt them out. . . . I am sorry that we cannot take them in the Home in any other way.[19]

Mrs. Thomasson quickly accepted the terms of South's offer and returned the completed indentures (which South had signed prior to forwarding) accompanied by a brief note.

> Just a few lines to thank you very much for your kindness in getting the Society to receive my children. I cannot express in words how grateful I am, and I pray to God that my children will be always happy under your care.[20]

For many of the women, the finality of a legal termination of guardianship distinguished their relationships with the VCAS from those that had prevailed with orphanages, extended families, and communities. The Thomasson case, however, is an affecting example of the contradictory nature of this legalistic, inflexible approach to child rescue. Mrs. Thomasson's letter, along with the completed indenture forms, arrived in the hands of her two children. Almost immediately, South wrote to their mother.

> The two little children arrived, but before I could possibly receive them into the Home as our wards, I want you to give me a little information. . . . Are the children Spanish, partly Indian, or partly colored. It is very important that I should know exactly the facts regarding their parentage and Nationality. I thought from your name, "[Thomasson]" the children would be swedish, but now I don't know what they are. Please let me know at once.[21]

South also wrote to Sergeant Graham of the Provincial Police in Kelowna inquiring about the background of the children who were now his wards. Graham responded,

> I have the honor to report as follows. . . . Mr. Thomasson was drowned in the Sask. River in 1918 while employed as a bridge builder, leaving Mrs. Thomasson with five children. Four of the

Children are in the children's home in Regina. . . . Mrs. Thomasson came here about 3 years ago . . . bringing her youngest child with her. The other child was born in Kelowna and she claims that a man named Norman Oakwood of this place is the father of the child. Oakwood seems to have given her some little money for awhile to help support the child but since the first of this year has given her nothing. . . . Mrs. Thomasson appears to me to be about half white and half indian so I guess that will account for the appearance of the children.[22]

The Thomasson case highlights one limitation of a child rescue strategy built around the termination of a birth parent's guardianship. Whether public guardianship was obtained by means of indenture or by apprehending the child, the VCAS had few options that would allow for the termination of its guardianship in favor of the birth parent. The indenture agreement contained no specific escape clauses, while the Children's Protection Act required that the Court or the Society determine that a return to parental guardianship would be "for the benefit of the child."

Child rescuers often pointed out that the newfound legal status granted them under child protection acts made them more effective at avoiding "imposture"—their term for the foisting of private responsibilites (in the form of children) upon the charity or the public purse—than orphanages and other forms of charitable aid had been. Equally able to subvert the impositions of financially irresponsible fathers, maternally irresponsible mothers, and racial and ethnic groups deemed incapable of fulfilling the obligations of full citizenship, the Society appeared well equipped to cultivate a citizenry built on a political foundation fractured by class, gender, and ethnicity.

The recourse to a quasi-criminal form of law in place of contractual agreements, which had previously governed nonfamilial forms of care for children, along with its reliance on judicial fact-finding, highlighted the unique public authority of the VCAS. They were elevated from providers of charity to administrators of justice. However, child rescuers were not alone in their recourse to justice. Correspondence housed in the Society's files illustrates that clients clearly understood the obligations that public status and, most important, the rule of law imposed upon the Society.

One of the larger families encountered in the present study consisted of seven children committed to the VCAS by a magistrate in

Grand Forks, initially due to nonsupport from their father. Shortly after their transfer to the Children's Home in Vancouver, their mother wrote to South requesting that the older children be permitted to write to her. Casting rather nebulous aspersions on her character, South suggested that it was in the children's best interests to sever all connections with her.

> You know Mrs. Gertz, they say some terrible things about your character, and how you can write to me and ask why the children are not allowed to correspond with you, I don't know. We want them to forget that they had a father and mother such as you are.[23]

Mrs. Gertz's reply to South, written one month later, is instructive. Obviously unclear about why her husband's nonsupport should render her a poor influence on her children, she argues for access to her children based not on her civil rights or the best interests of the children, but on her record as a solid, long-suffering wife and mother.

> I can't see where I have not done fair by Mr. Gertz. . . . I have worked away from home to help take care of the children. . . . Now you are aware that it is some work for a woman to wash, make and mend for that many children without [having to work] away from home but I couldn't see them go hungry as they would of done if I had not. . . . We had got down so there wasn't hardly anything in the house to eat but potatoes and flour enough to last two days and I asked him to see about getting something and he said why did he half to russell and I said if he did not I would half to, so he said alright, they could get along without me. . . . Now if I am unfair with Mr. Gertz I would like to know in which way.[24]

Mrs. Gertz's attempts did not ultimately address South's concerns. Explaining that he had only broached the nature of his concerns to protect her, he outlined the source and nature of the complaints against Mrs. Gertz.

> Now to show you the fix I am in—I have tried as far as I can to protect you, but I was speaking to a lady the other day about your baby, and she came from Grand Forks, but I did not know that. She seemed very nice and she said, "No, not the Gertz

baby, no thank you; I am told that it's mother does not know who his father is. . . . I understand from several others who were there, that you are not living right with your husband that is to say, you are doing wrong with men, and that is what I want answered.[25]

Mrs. Gertz's response to these accusations is reproduced here at length.

> Now you say that you are told that I do not know who the children's father is. Well I can safely tell you that Mr. Gertz is the father of my seven children. . . . I have been a true wife to Mr. Gertz the 18 years we have been married. . . . You know that the law in Canada is that a man is supposed to support his wife and family but they failed to make Mr. Gertz. They have left him go so he can go and get another wife and bring some more children into the world and when she won't slave for him no longer he can take the children away from her as he has done me and go for another fresh start. . . . There have not been anything proven about my character and you are going on hearsay and you are some man of law to go on hearsay. You say those children was good and pure minded, who brought them up that way it was not *you*. . . . It seems as if Mr. Gertz can do anything. He is like yourself, a gentleman, privileged character to do and say as he like.[26]

Mrs. Gertz's plea in the face of her nameless accusers is eloquent testimony of the resistance which, on occasion, confronted Charles South. In her spirited defense of her own conduct, her pride in her children, and her refusal to wither before the legal authority commanded by South, Mrs. Gertz provides an important counterpoint for some of the earlier cases examined here, in which the case files recorded only resignation.

More specifically, Mrs. Gertz's letter illustrates the variety of bases around which clients shaped the claims that they advanced toward the VCAS. Mrs. Gertz's claims reflect a recognition that any consideration granted by South would hinge on her role as wife and mother. Initially, she defends herself as a "true wife" and urges "for the sake of her children" that South disclose the source of his information.

Ultimately, however, Gertz goes beyond claims based on her gender-specific role to protest the inequity confronting her and her children. The power of her words arises from her penetration of the gendered nature of the laws and agencies to which she refers. Her own experiences are harnessed to illustrate the gendered nature of the privileges and obligations of fathers and mothers.

Finally, in chastising South as "some man of law," Gertz highlights the contradictory nature of the public, legal authority of children's aid societies. For all its organizational benefits, this public identity also imposed obligations on the Society to be governed by the rule of law in a way that contractually based, private, charitable orphanages had not been compelled. A final case closes this chapter by extending this logic. For some clients, the distinction between charity and justice so vehemently traced by child rescuers had a direct impact on the basis of their claims upon the Society.

As Fraser (1989, 1990) and Fraser and Gordon (1994) argue, activists and policymakers have historically advanced three types of claims for assistance: needs, entitlements, and rights. The cases examined earlier illustrate that most men approaching the VCAS saw care and education as an entitlement premised on their financial support. Although some women approached the Society with similar expectations, their overtures were, in the majority of cases, converted into claims based on needs. As dependent members of the private sphere, both women and children were regarded as essentially needy, in contrast to the independence and self-sufficiency of (male) citizens.

Increasingly throughout the late nineteenth and early twentieth centuries, these claims were transposed, first by activists and reformers and later, as documented here, by claimants themselves into the language of rights. In the case files of the VCAS, evidence is left by women who approached public institutions seeking justice, not charity, for themselves and their children. However, these expressions of resistance often drew upon a gendered conception of rights, which reflected important elements of the fractured forms of citizenship underlying the practice of child rescue. As Gwendolyn Mink notes, "welfare fastened worthy women's citizenship to domestic motherhood . . . [w]ithholding the tools of independent citizenship from most women" (1994, p. 118).

When Mrs. Shore initially approached the VCAS in January 1912, having been deserted by her husband, South offered only to aid in finding employment for her eldest son. Her response to South's offer was an eloquent expression of the rights to which she felt entitled and an illustration of her appreciation of the leverages she commanded in her request for public support for herself and her children.

> Clare [her fifteen-year-old son] went to the plumbing shop which you referred him too. Said he did not need anyone at present, but might need some one later on. He has the promise of several places when the work begins, but promises does not keep the life in anyone. . . . Now if the law will not protect these children as it should while I am with them and willing to take care of them, I shall have to leave them; not because I want to but because I have to. I cannot endure seeing them want for things they need. I am behind with the rent and other things thro no fault of mine. . . . I know that you have done your best concerning the matter, but then there must be something definite done and that very soon. If the law will not take [my husband] in hand and make him do his duty toward the children, then the law will have to provide for them. . . . Do not take up any charity collections for me. I do not want charity, only justice.[27]

Although many lone fathers regarded the Society as little more than a boarding school, women left to care for their children alone tended to equate the Society with the law (Adamoski, 1995). They drew a clear connection between the Society and the various legal provisions that presumably created obligations for their husbands. They recognized their own inequitable position before the law, but they showed little reluctance toward framing their claims in the language of rights and justice.

The rights and obligations upon which these women focused were based upon positions in the private sphere. For both women, the primary claim was advanced on behalf of their children, toward whom their father bore a duty of support. The forms of resistance utilized by women such as Gertz and Shore reflect the nature of these imposed rights. Although they protested the practical day-to-day inequities that they suffered as women, and although they utilized the language of rights to express their claims, they ultimately advanced their claims as mothers concerned to protect the rights of their children. Their arguments resonated with the maternal feminism that constituted one important strand of the feminist movement in Western democracies in the early twentieth century.

Ultimately, the majority of women who approached the Society with dependent children were unable to access forms of aid that would permit them the same degree of independence allowed for fathers. Barbara Nelson has described the "agony and fury" felt by lone mothers at the turn of the century—women who were forced to accept "that they might have to lose their children in order to support them" (1990, p. 28). Those emotions are palpable in the cases examined here. The VCAS case files furnish a moving account of the statutory resources and daily practices of the Society as an "arena of struggle"—a public, legalized form of child care that created at least some limited opportunities for women and children (Bartholomew & Hunt, 1990, p. 51). This contention is supported by the frequency with which parents resorted to the Society and by their ability to carve options, however distasteful, from the available resources.

As we pass from the early twentieth century to the present, the relationship between the Canadian state and its citizenry is undergoing significant shifts. Globalizing economic forces and the "North American security perimeter" have fundamentally assaulted the nationalistic vision that infused the foundations of the Canadian welfare state. As Canadian citizens are increasingly reduced to economic actors, the discriminatory forms of citizenship outlined previously have returned with a particular vengeance.

Today, the invisibility of "family work"—that tenuous basis upon which the mothers portrayed here made claims for public support—handicaps mothers raising children alone even more significantly than it did in earlier decades. Labeled nonproductive in the era of the entrepreneurial citizen (Brodie, 2002), these women and their children have born the brunt of welfare state retraction. Today, Canadian women raising children apart from their fathers shoulder not only their so-called natural duties as mothers but the obligations of workers as well. Of course, as exemplified in the previous cases, recourse of mothers to paid work is not new. However, the portrayal of lone parenthood as a condemnable lifestyle choice has justified uniquely punitive social policy reforms throughout North America, with predictable victims (Solinger, 1998). In 1997, more than one-half of Canadian lone-parent families headed by women had incomes below the low-income cutoff, (Statistics Canada, 2000). Behind these statistics lie lived experiences and desperate choices similar to those described earlier in this chapter. It appears inevitable that many Canadian women will still be forced to confront the unnatural option of living apart from their children.

NOTES

1. Add. MSS. 672, vol. 174. Letter from South to Manager of Laurential Milk Co. requesting a donation of milk after death of the Home's cow. Dated January 21, 1914.

2. Case number 322. Running record dated September 1925 and August 1928. Case numbers are derived from a coding scheme designed to protect the identity of the Society's clients. Researchers granted access to this collection may contact the author for a key. Pseudonyms are used throughout this chapter when referring to clients of the Vancouver Children's Aid Society.

3. Case number 2003. Letter from A. M. Stephens to R. Grayston (Superintendent-Secretary), September 4, 1924. Emphasis in original.

4. Case number 2003. Statement of Grayston, Sept. 20, 1924.

5. Add. MSS 672, Vol. 129, *Annual Report of the Vancouver Children's Aid Society* (Hereinafter, *Annual Report*) 1911, p. 29.

6. Cited in *Annual Report* 1939, p. 6.

7. Case number 490201. Apparently a press release written by South, c. 1913.

8. Case number 2811. Court Transcript, Report of Officer Lowry, September 17, 1913.

9. Case number 2811. Letter found with child. Circa September 13, 1913.

10. Case number 1110. Letter from Chief Constable to South, August 20, 1909.

11. Case number 1907. Letter to South from Rev. R. M. Thompson, February 23, 1912.

12. Add. MSS. 672, vol. 147. Letter from Rev. C. Ladner of Kamloops to South dated October 9, 1913.

13. Add. MSS. 672, vol. 147. Letter from South to Rev. C. Ladner of Kamloops dated October 24, 1913.

14. Case number 0212. Letter from South to Minister in Nanaimo dated August 27, 1914.

15. Case number 0212. Letter from mother to South dated March 15, 1915.

16. Case number 0213. Letter from South to adoptive father dated Febrary 1, 1915.

17. Case number 0212. Letter from South to mother dated July 16, 1915.

18. Case number 1624. Letter from Mother to South, May 23, 1921.

19. Case number 1624. Reply from South to Mother, June 1, 1921.

20. Case number 1624. Letter from Mother to South, July 11, 1921.

21. Case number 1624. Letter from South to Mother, July 18, 1921.

22. Case number 1624. Letter from Graham of the Provincial Police, Kelowna to South, July 28, 1921.

23. Case number 0707. South to Mother, Febrary 15, 1922.

24. Case number 0707. Mother to South, March 14, 1922.

25. Case number 0707. South to Mother, March 18, 1922.
26. Case number 0707. Mother to South, May 1, 1922.
27. Case number 1216. Letter from mother to South, dated January 29, 1912.

REFERENCES

Adamoski, R. (1995). *Their duties toward the children: Citizenship and the practice of child rescue in early twentieth century British Columbia.* Unpublished doctoral dissertation, Simon Fraser University, Vancouver, BC.

Adamoski, R. (2002). Charity is one thing and the administration of justice is another: Law and the politics of familial regulation in early twentieth century B.C. In J. McLaren, R. Menzies, & D. E. Chunn (Eds.), *Regulating lives: Social control, law and the state in British Columbia history* (pp. 145-169). Vancouver, BC: UBC Press.

Bartholomew, A. & Hunt, A. (1990). What's wrong with rights? *Journal of Law and Inequality, 9,* 1-58.

Bradbury, B. (1993). *Working families: Age, gender, and daily survival in industrializing Montreal.* Toronto, ON: McClelland and Stewart Inc.

Brodie, J. (2002). Three stories of Canadian citizenship. In R. Adamoski, D. Chunn, & R. Menzies, (Eds.), *Contesting Canadian citizenship: Historical readings* (pp. 43-60). Peterborough, ON: Broadview Press.

Fraser, N. (1989). *Unruly practices: Power, discourse and gender in contemporary social theory.* Minneapolis: University of Minnesota Press.

Fraser, N. (1990). Struggle over needs: Outline of a socialist-feminist critical theory of late capitalist political culture. In L. Gordon (Ed.), *Women, the state, and welfare* (pp. 199-225). Madison: University of Wisconsin Press.

Fraser, N. & Gordon, L. (1994). Civil citizenship against social citizenship? In B. van Steenbergen (Ed.), *The condition of citizenship* (pp. 90-107). London: Sage.

Kealey, L. (1979). (Ed.). *A not unreasonable claim: Women and reform in Canada, 1880s-1920s.* Toronto, ON: Canadian Women's Educational Press.

Koven, S. & Michel, S. (1993). (Eds.). *Mothers of a new world: Maternalist politics and the origins of welfare states.* London: Routledge.

Mink, G. (1994). Welfare reform in historical perspective, *Social Justice 21*(1), 114-131.

Mink, G. (2001). Violating women: Rights abuses in the welfare police state, *Annals of the American Academy of Politica and Social Science, 577,* 79-93.

Nelson, B. (1990). The origins of the two-channel welfare state: Workmen's compensation and mother's aid. In L. Gordon (Ed.), *Women, the state, and welfare* (pp. 123-151). Madison: University of Wisconsin Press.

Orloff, A. (1993). Gender and the social rights of citizenship: The comparative analysis of gender relations and welfare states. *American Sociological Review, 58,* 303-328.

Solinger, R. (1998). Dependency and choice: The two faces of Eve. *Social Justice* *25*(1), 1-27.

Statistics Canada. (2000). *Women in Canada 2000: A gender based statistical report.* Catalogue number 89-503-XPE.

Chapter 8

Missing Mothers in a Mother-Centered World: Adolescent Girls Growing Up in Kinship Care

Deborah Connolly Youngblood

Savannah is fifteen years old. Since she was four days old, she has lived with her grandmother who has been her primary caregiver. She knows her mother, whom she has seen sporadically throughout her life. During one visit her mother asked Savannah how she felt about her. Savannah replied,

> I don't know you and I don't like you. I don't care too much for you . . . I don't ever want to get to know you . . . You know you can never change.

Reportedly, Savannah's mother was angered and hurt by this response and Savannah was forced to apologize. Why would Savannah's mother ask such a question of her daughter? Is she looking for reassurance of daughterly love? Is she hoping to relieve her own guilt or ambivalence about not having raised her child? Is she looking for a motherly identity through acceptance from her daughter? Or did she really want the truth, even if it hurt?

Missing mothers or mothers who live apart from their children are a socially marginalized and demonized group. According to dominant Western cultural characterizations, mothers are expected to love, nurture, and provide primary care for their children. This normative image of the good mother is narrowly circumscribed even though women who give birth to children are a widely diverse group. It should not be surprising that many women who have children are unable to inhabit the conventional model, yet we are surprised, shocked, and even offended when mothers live apart from their children. Perhaps rather than investigating the individual mothers who deviate from the norm—as we seem inclined to do—we should investigate the norms themselves and think about the effects they have on women, men, and children.

The emphasis on the role of the mother may place undue burdens on the relationship between mothers and children. My previous work and the work of others (Connolly, 2000a; Ladd-Taylor & Umansky, 1998; Ragoné & Twine, 2000; Tsing, 1990), explores how the over-wrought idealization of the good mother stigmatizes women whose circumstances make it an impossible standard to pursue. I argue that although the good mother model is purported to be class and race neutral, it actually represents a set of circumstances that require substantial resources and reflect parenting practices espoused primarily in white, middle-class culture. Thus, women who do not fit this narrow category often find themselves judged as bad or unfit mothers.

This scenario is further exacerbated by the biologizing of the mother-child bond—the dominant belief that motherlove, and therefore good mothering, is built in to women's nature. The naturalization of good motherhood means that when women fall short of the model, they are viewed as failed women as well as failed mothers (Connolly, 2000a, 2000b). Since the good mother model implicitly demands an affluent background, low-income women (many of whom are women of color) are more likely to bear the brunt of negative judgments against them.

My current research on adolescent girls growing up in kinship care explores how children, too, are emotionally burdened by the good mother model. I contend that young people would struggle less with a sense that something is wrong in their lives, indeed wrong with them, if the dominant Western paradigms that idealize motherhood were adjusted to provide for more diversity in child raising.

Kinship care refers to a familial arrangement in which a relative other than the biological parent is raising a child. Some researchers suggest that the prevalence of kinship care among African-American communities has lessened the stigmatization, creating an alternative norm that accepts diverse caregivers rather than focusing on the biological mother (Stack, 1974; Crosbie-Burnett & Lewis, 1999). In her research on childkeeping in a low-income African-American community, Stack (1974) suggests that kinship care is not only an alternative strategy for child rearing but also an implicit critique of dominant ideologies of the nuclear family. A larger comparative study of African-American and Anglo-American youth being raised by relatives would be required to determine if African-American teens feel more comfortable with their family status than their Anglo-American peers. However, my research suggests, at least preliminarily, that African-American adolescent girls feel a definite sense of loss when they are raised apart from their birth mothers, and this experience appears to be only minimally mediated by the greater acceptance of diverse family arrangements among this population.

This chapter focuses particularly on the relationships between missing mothers and daughters. According to the dominant paradigm, mothers are expected to provide their daughters with a role model mediated by a powerful emotional bond between them. Although boys are supposed to grow apart from their mothers, building masculine identities as they move into adolescence, girls are expected to maintain strong identifications. These identifications often result in volatile teenage years in traditional or white middle-class families, as adolescent girls seek independence. However, the turmoil itself is seen as a developmental stage. That is, there is *supposed* to be a mother to rebel against. Although growing up apart from the day-to-day care of a birth mother certainly has strong effects on boys and girls of all ages, I focus here on the experiences of African-American adolescent girls between the ages of eleven and twenty.

This study is based on qualitative research conducted in the San Francisco Bay Area at Edgewood Center for Children and Families Institute for the Study of Community-Based Services. To help me design and conduct open-ended interviews for the study, I hired three adolescent girls, two African-American and one Latina, between the ages of fifteen and twenty who had personal experience living in kinship care. I spent several months training them in research skills and interview techniques. My hope was that adolescents would be able to open doors with other teens that are often closed to adult interviewers such as myself. The findings presented in this chapter are based on twenty-five open-ended interviews conducted by the youth researchers and me.

MISSING MOTHERS

On January 1, 2001, the headline of *The Examiner* in San Francisco read, "Alternative to dumping newborns: New law allows infants to be left at hospital, no questions asked." This new state legislation gives mothers a window of seventy-two hours in which they may
anonymously leave newborns at a hospital. It was created to guard
against "women leaving their infants to die in dumpsters or alley-
ways" (p. A1). The law is designed to support women who give birth
to offspring but who do not conform to normative expectations of
nurturing their babies. This law suggests a kind of social softening toward these women. They are given an escape route from a mothering
role they either cannot or do not want to accept, with no punitive
strings attached. I support this legislation in that it moves toward de-
criminalizing women who feel, usually with a sense of desperation,
that they are unable to keep a child.

Even though I am in favor of this legislation, it is based upon and
reinforces a dominant Western belief about parental rights and responsibilities: mothers have exclusive responsibility for their offspring. The law allows women to maintain anonymity when dropping
off infants and then gives them two weeks to change their minds before maternal rights are terminated and the child can be adopted. No
provisions are noted for paternal rights and responsibilities.

This legislation makes concrete what is already true in practice.
Only the mother is truly significant; only the mother is truly responsible for the child. That conservative groups such as the National Right
to Life Committee and liberal groups such as Planned Parenthood
both support this law suggests that people at both ends of the political
spectrum agree on the primacy of the mother in relation to biological
children. Fathers are peripheral. A dedicated father tends to be committed first to the mother and then, because of that conjugal connection, becomes connected to the child. This legislation reinforces the
belief that impregnating fathers are naturally or normally more de-
tached from the children they help create. While impregnating is
viewed as primarily a sexual act, birthing is the maternal act to which
is attached the primary rights, responsibilities, burdens, and weights
of parenthood.

Although fathers are not expected to prioritize their children above
all else, mothers are. When they do not, they are demonized (Con-

nolly, 2000a; Ladd-Taylor & Umansky, 1998; Tsing, 1990). A woman who gives her child to relatives may be regarded as irresponsible or selfish. A woman whose child is removed by child welfare authorities and then fails to regain custody because she does not follow the rules, for example, by failing to complete drug treatment, is thought of as not simply irresponsible but selfish, cold, even inhuman. Women are expected to sacrifice for their children. They are expected to place them above all else in their lives. Consider how Savannah criticizes her biological mother.

> She is always putting men before her children. I've always hated that, always. And she still does it, like her husband is like the number one priority and I have to please him. . . . I ain't gonna let no man run over me and he ain't gonna take over my life. . . . I don't care how long you've been with a man; you're always supposed to put your children before you put that man. I'm just saying once you have something that was inside of you for nine months and you carried, it's like you're going to *know* [emphasis in original] that person. You're never supposed to put a man, husband, I don't care who it is, before your children. It's like, you just don't do that. It's like blood first, then your marriage.

Savannah's critique of her mother provokes empathy. It seems understandable that a daughter who feels rejected by her mother and given less priority than the men in her mother's life would feel angry and hurt. While not diminishing the legitimacy of Savannah's pain, I do want to explore the way she calls on a biological model to criticize her mother's behavior toward her. That Savannah was carried within her mother's body for nine months means that they "know" each other in a deep way unavailable to her mother's male partners: "blood first, then your marriage."

The biological model that reveres motherhood and the mother-child bond is one of the major stumbling blocks for missing mothers and children such as Savannah. When a social-biological phenomenon, such as motherly love, is scripted as purely natural, then those individuals whose lives do not match the norm become socially ostracized and experience internal conflict. For example, consider this dialogue between Larissa, who is growing up in kinship care, and Tina, a peer interviewer.

TINA: So your mom's drug use and stuff, how does that affect your life now?

LARISSA: It don't 'cause I don't go see her.

TINA: You don't want to see your mom?

LARISSA: Nope.

TINA: Do you love your mom?

LARISSA: Nope.

TINA: So, you don't have any relationship with your mother at all?

LARISSA: None.

It is jarring to hear Larissa talk about her missing mother this way, particularly hearing the absence of affect in her voice. Such discomfort tells us something about ourselves as well as her. It reveals the mandate for mother-child relationships to be close and primary. Even though the mother-child bond is challenged here—the prominence of the mother in the girl's life is not. Although Larissa reports that she neither has nor wants a relationship with her mother, her words throughout the interview suggest that the absence of the mother-child relationship deeply affects her life. Tina, her peer interviewer, described this phenomenon in this way:

> I noticed that pretty much all the interviews that I did, they just gave like the same breezy answers: "I don't care. I can't stand her. I hate her." It was either the hate, "I want nothing to do with her," or it was "We still have a good relationship and, you know, I don't worry about it because it's the past." I think that even though they gave me that flat out answer, it wasn't the whole truth because you can't have the "I hate" without the "I'm hurt." And I think that "I'm hurt" always came first in both answers.

Tina points to a subtext in the straightforward responses to questions about missing mothers. She notes that whether the description of the mother-child relationship is positive or negative, a pain caused by a sense of rejection and confusion underpins the relationship. Just as mothers who raise their children have an enormous impact on their children's lives, mothers who do not raise their children also have a strong influence. However, we must ask how much of that impact is inevitable and how much of it is produced by cultural ideologies of what mother-child relationships are supposed to be? What would it take to shift the cultural paradigms that characterize biological motherhood and alleviate the pressure for mother-child relationships to be uniformly primary?

THE ADOLESCENT CODE OF SILENCE

Adolescent girls with missing mothers, whose sense of self is developed in a culture that reveres the mother-child relationship and questions any arrangement that falls outside its confines, struggle to find a sense of self-legitimacy. Savannah, for example, recalls confiding in a friend that the reason her grandmother is raising her is because her mother is addicted to crack cocaine. Her friend revealed this to others, and Savannah soon found herself the object of taunts from schoolmates who called her "crack baby" and stupid.

The bad mother category of women who use drugs during pregnancy stigmatizes not only women but their children as well. Savannah's peers are responding to the cultural notion that we deserve the lot we are born into, and the lot we are born into is tied more closely to the circumstances of the mother than anything else. Savannah has none of the characteristics associated with fetal exposure to drugs, but she faces people judging her both as physically imperfect because of that exposure and as socially questionable because of her birth mother. Savannah learned that her family life does not measure up to the social norm and to avoid being taunted she must be vigilant about not telling other people "her business," as she puts it.

Many youth in kinship care feel stigmatized culturally and conflicted internally by the absence of their mothers, and they also find it hard to devise strategies to minimize this effect. Teenagers may be particularly invested in concealing not only their wounds but also the very existence of their differences. Adolescence is a time of intense peer comparison, when social codes are stringently defined and youth who are unable to fit in with their peers are often bullied and ostracized. Based on my experience working with youth, young people absorb cultural ideologies without the reflection and critique that sometimes help buffer adults, so they may perceive their anomalies as more severe and isolating.

Take, for example, Jody, a teen who invited her nonresidential mother to her church choir performance and then was horrified and ashamed when her mother attended visibly high on crack cocaine. This teenager's shame stems from her sense that her mother's behavior is a reflection of her and that people will judge her accordingly. And that may be true, particularly among adolescent peers. A more secure adult may be able to individuate from her mother, but, for the most part, teenagers' main strategies are to deny and conceal the parts of their lives that deviate from social norms.

Another version of these denial strategies is exemplified by Brianna, a fifteen-year-old girl who kept insisting during her interview that her family life is really like a fairy tale:

> I had an absolutely perfect childhood . . . like a twenty-first [century] *Leave It to Beaver* type of family. I still call my momma "ma'am." When she asks something I be like, "Yes, ma'am. No, ma'am." I mean it's cool. I like it.

She fails to mention here that her "momma" is really her maternal aunt. She was removed from the care of her birth mother because of her mother's drug abuse. Her life is not quite as traditional as she would have us believe. One wonders whether she lives the fairy tale existence she presents or whether she has developed this story for public consumption.

Whether an adolescent girl creates an alternative reality or conceals a difficult truth, it is a complicated task for her to craft a conventional public persona while living something else. The majority of girls did this by maintaining an unusually high level of privacy. Many of them talk about never having friends over to their house, or only inviting a select few who "know the deal." Many of the youth said that they had very few friends and referred instead to having "associates." Associates, the girls explained, are people one knows and is friendly with at school or other activities but they are not people with whom to share personal experiences. As the girls put it, they are not people "you tell your business to." As sixteen-year-old Miranda explains,

> Associates are kinda like a work relationship. You only talk to them about, you know, how most work relationships are. "Hi, how are you?" and it never goes past that . . . I mean you can go out with them and do fun things with them but you never go too personal.

Many girls had no one with whom they discussed their family life. Those who did had just one or two people in whom they confided, and these confidantes were almost always in similar family situations.

Another sign that these teenagers feel alone is their expression of the need to be strong and responsible for themselves and others. On numerous occasions when asked the question, "What advice would you give to a child who was going through the same things that you have in your life," their answers were some version of, "Help your mom and don't give her a hard time." This suggests that these adolescents see themselves as having control over their mothers' inability to care for them and that perhaps if they had just been better daughters, their mothers would not have needed to leave. This self-blaming may increase the youths' sense that they must hide their real selves and maintain a strong public front, pretending that everything is fine all the time.

Children in kinship care are often torn between feeling loyalty to their mothers and trying to survive in a setting where they were not being adequately cared for. This bind is wrenching enough without adding on the belief that they are partially responsible. One can easily understand how a child who has been removed from her mother's care might reflect and imagine that if only she herself had tried harder—everything would have been different.

Some adolescent girls want to conceal the difficult truths in their lives from themselves as well as outsiders. When asked about the past, many of them replied that they tried not to think about it. Some of them tried to fill up their lives with other activities, keeping themselves busy so that they would not dwell on family issues. Miranda put it this way:

> That's why I'm always into all this stuff, you know—job, school, show choir, ILS [Independent Living Skills], all this other stuff—keep my mind busy so I don't have time to think about it. But when I do think about it, of course I'll probably shed like a tear or two and think, "Why me? Why is my family not perfect like everybody else's?" But then when I come to realize, it's like, everybody's family got some false teeth.

Perhaps one of the ways that adolescent girls recognize that many people live in families quite different from the dominant Western image of the family is through involvement with relevant support groups. As Miranda notes, she participates in the Independent Living Skills class, an activity for teens growing up in kinship care offered by the Edgewood Center. The class is designed to prepare young people to live independently after the age of eighteen. For some teenagers, this was the only arena in which they could relax and drop their pretenses. Here they see that others are growing up with missing mothers too and that no judgment is passed on that fact. For adolescent girls who are coping with the fear of being revealed as Other, such a safe space is critical.

MOTHERS WHO ARE MISSED

During a discussion of family in one Independent Living Skills class that I attended, youth in kinship care expressed repeatedly and with intensity that their birth mothers "owed them an explanation." These youth wanted some kind of a reason to explain why their mothers did not raise them. As Kara puts it:

It made me feel bad and ask questions like, "Why did you give me up? You didn't even give me a chance to prove that I'm good enough for you."

One reason these youth may feel particularly rejected is because of the cultural doctrines that identify blood relations as representing the epitome of nurturance and emotional closeness. Indeed, these doctrines lead children living apart from their mothers to pose the frequently asked question, "Why didn't she keep me?" (Burlingham-Brown, 1994). Although such questions seem to well up from the inner emotional workings of a hurt child, at least one researcher points out that in some cultures in which adoption is more common such questions are not commonly posed by adopted children (Gailey, 2000). Hence, we must address the possibility that American children in kinship care are not victims of their mother's imperfections as much as they are victims of a cultural doctrine that does not offer them a positive framework to affirm their familial arrangements.

Consider again Savannah, who lives in the care of her grandmother. Savannah's mother has been in and out of her life, sporadically calling but often refusing to reveal where she was living. Sometimes, Savannah's mother would show up unexpectedly for events such as Savannah's graduation from eighth grade or her brother's graduation from high school. These surprise visits were hard on Savannah. She must negotiate a mother-child relationship that does not fit any of the traditional categories. Savannah says it this way:

You know I try to give her respect, but it's some of the things she does that, like, really irks me. She tries to tell me how to dress and it gets on my nerves. In the cold she tells me to wear two shirts and a puff coat, and it doesn't get that cold in San Francisco to wear all of that. You know in Arizona it might be like that . . . but I was like, it's not like that out here. You never dressed me before; why are you trying to dress me now?

Savannah conveys her contradictory situation well. She tries to accord her mother due respect, but has a hard time doing so when her mother has not earned it. Should she defer to a woman based solely on their biological connection? Is she expected to *feel* respectful toward her mother regardless of their history together? For Savannah, the social obligation to show and feel maternal respect is emotionally messy. Savannah is torn between the social pressure to respect her birth mother and the evidence that her mother is not, in fact, behaving like a mother. Savannah sums up her anger and conflicted feelings by pointing out the hypocrisy in her mother's presumption that she has the right to tell Savannah what to wear, even though she has taken no responsibility for dressing Savannah in the past, when she really needed someone to dress her. Savannah is asserting newfound competencies even while pointing to the missing mother whose absence still haunts her.

Here the mother-child negotiations are burdened by the naturalized expectations of what Savannah allegedly should have received from her mother and how the two should feel about each other. Similar to other teenage girls moving through normal stages of adolescent rebellion, Savannah's struggle for greater independence has an additional conflict. Although she wants to establish herself as separate from her mother, she never experienced the prior enmeshment with her mother that is typical among girls raised by their birth mothers. Kinship care provides Savannah with a stable home, but she cannot escape the confusion stemming from the cultural norm of the good mother.

Denise also struggles to understand why her mother is missing from her life. Consider her description of how she came to live with her grandmother.

> Well, my two older sisters and I, we all lived with her because, um, my mom was like, she would rather party and hang out with people and she would, like, drop us at my grandmother's house anyway all the time. And she would never have any food in the house and have strange people in the house and she [grandmother] just took over guardianship.

This youth sees her living arrangement with her grandmother—even though it may be nurturing—as marred by the fact that she ended up there by default, deserted by a mother who would rather party than care for her children.

Missing mothers need to be understood within a larger social context that does not condone abuse and neglect but that recognizes the wider social pressures, discriminations, and obstacles that significantly challenge women trying unsuccessfully to raise their children (Murphy & Rosenbaum, 1999; Connolly, 2000a, 2000b). We cannot expect these children to have this understanding as long as we live in a culture that lacks it. These girls are frequently left to sift through a painful rejection with little social support or understanding. They are left to cope with two absences: the absence of their mother and the absence of cultural resources to treat children reared apart from their birth mothers as a regular part of life itself.

Tracy, a nineteen-year-old woman in kinship care, describes to an interviewer, Isabel, her relationship with her mother this way:

TRACY: My relationship with my mom was strange because I never really seen her, so ummm, I'd see her in and out but basically my relationship was with my little sister and brothers I had to take care of . . .

ISABEL: So you were in more of a mother role?

TRACY: A mother role, yeah.

ISABEL: So what do you appreciate most about your family?

TRACY: Well, I appreciate my mother because of all it took for my mom to go out and change, you know what I'm saying? She attended a five-year program . . . one of those rehab homes . . . I appreciate that she did because I had too much things to do. I felt alone, and if she could get my sister and brothers back, then she could be a mother to them.

ISABEL: So who do you think has been the most influential person in your life? Who has made the most impact?

TRACY: My mother.

ISABEL: Why?

TRACY: Because I want her to improve.

ISABEL: So do you think your life has been different because of your mother?

TRACY: Yeah, because I am determined to have things in my life. I put a lot of pressure on me, because I don't want to be like my mom.

The contradictions Tracy displays here are striking. Every question asked of her is answered in relation to her mother, even though she starts out by telling the interviewer that her mother is someone she has "never really seen." In spite of this absence, she acknowledges her mother as the person she appreciates the most, who has had the greatest influence on her life, and who has made her life different because of her actions. Why does Tracy's mother provide the center point from which everything stems and to which it returns? Why does this woman who did not raise her and did not live with her persist as the foundation, albeit cracked and shaky, on which Tracy sees the rest of her life resting? How might we alter the singular concentration of parental responsibility upon mothers to relax these intense pressures that are then experienced by everyone involved? How can we best support young people whose mothers are unable or unwilling to raise them, instilling in them a positive sense of self and a sense of family unity that is not dependent upon being raised by a competent and loving birth mother?

NATURALIZING SOCIAL POLICY

The cultural priorities of blood relations, family preservation, and family autonomy create the underpinnings for our social policies on child welfare (Bartholet, 1999). In spite of significant diversity in the composition of family-like groups, a limited definition of the family still persists—a definition that treats traditional heterosexual marriage and biological offspring as the paradigm of the legitimate family (Coontz, 1992). Numerous constituencies find themselves shuffled outside this cultural definition, including adoptive families, gay and lesbian families, homeless families, stepfamilies, foster families, and kinship care families. Increasing numbers of children find themselves in one or more of these situations.

The history of prioritizing bloodlines can be traced back to the European roots of the white American culture. The protection of social standing and legitimacy required strict monitoring of biological lineage. The dominant, contemporary American paradigm of liberalism and meritocracy blurs the way class divisions are largely inherited. Therefore, bloodlines, which once symbolized a family's social standing and legitimacy, now symbolize closeness and loyalty as proxies for love and bonding (Schneider, 1968). We no longer talk about protecting family sanctity so that there is no disruption of, say, the royal family line. Instead, we talk about preserving birth families because of their natural connectedness. Family policies assert a strong connection between sharing genetic material and sharing a deep emotional bond. However, just below the surface are distinctions about legitimacy and normality still contingent on biological relationships. Furthermore, perhaps we naturalize or biologize the family paradigm more intensely to cover up the actual pluralization of circumstances in which children are raised.

Contemporary American families are now viewed more narrowly, with an almost exclusive focus on the nuclear family. Indeed, as American families have become more mobile, the cultural emphasis on extended family has decreased. As divorce rates rise, women are overwhelmingly the head of lone-parent families. The ideal of motherhood becomes intensified even while many mothers are disconnected from a host of practical supports, as evidenced by the large number of mothers living in poverty, living without mates, exposed to violence, and living in unsafe conditions (Gordon, 1994; Polakow, 1993; Sidel, 1992).

The mother-child bond paradigm continues to gain strength in the United States. It is becoming increasingly institutionalized through legal rulings, medical practices, and child welfare policies. For example, Elizabeth Bartholet (1999) cites the case of "Baby Jessica" to illustrate the cultural priority of biological bonds over social bonds. In this case, the infant was placed with the family who wanted to adopt her shortly after the infant's birth when the birth mother relinquished her parental rights. Shortly thereafter, the birth mother changed her mind and was joined by the biological father who had not relinquished his parental rights at the time of adoption (as he had not been identified). Together they initiated legal proceedings to have Jessica returned to their care. After two and a half years, the courts ordered "Baby Jessica" be removed from the family she knew and placed with her biological parents. News coverage showed Jessica looking back toward her home and shrieking "Mommy!" as she was taken away to live with birth parents she had never known.

Baby Jessica is a complex case, but it exposes the strong priority placed on biology. Basically, while Jessica calls out for her (non-blood-related) mommy, the court uses biological evidence to tell her she is wrong. The act of mothering provided by her adoptive mother is superseded by the fact of biological production.

CONCLUSION

Kinship care is becoming an increasingly popular option in child welfare circles (Cox, 2000; Crumbley & Little, 1997; Gleeson & Hairston, 1999; Hegar & Scannapieco, 1999). Proponents see kinship care as a way of providing children with continuity and the maintenance of family ties, links to community and neighborhood, and a more consistent and permanent placement for children than nonrelative foster care. Critics claim that kinship care often places children in less than optimal homes, within families where previous abuse and/or neglect is likely to have taken place (presumably of the child's parents), and where children are less likely to be restricted from the parent who lost parental rights because of abuse and/or neglect. Bartholet (1999) and other critics promote the faster termination of an abusive parent's parental rights and the placement of children in permanent adoptive homes.

Both sides of the argument miss an important point. In foster care, kinship care, and adoptive homes children frequently experience a strong sense of mother loss. Although child safety and well-being need to be the primary points of immediate intervention in our work . with young people, a wider social context needs to be brought into focus. We must begin disrupting the idealizations of birth mothers that place all the responsibility for love and care on individual (under-resourced and fallible) women. We must begin promoting understandings of families as diverse groups that provide love, care, and nurturing. Together these shifts may allow young women growing up in a variety of family structures to find more outside acceptance and more inner peace. The singular nature of our vision of motherhood does not sit well with the lived world in which a plurality of modes of childrearing form a regular part of cultural life. This image is not only at odds with the world but also imposes a variety of injuries on the many children whose mode of rearing differs from a norm itself in need of pluralization.

One way to lessen the pain experienced by children growing up without their mothers, indeed the pain experienced by all members of nontraditional families, is to expand definitions of the family and emphasize social relations alongside biological ones. For instance, schools can begin teaching about diverse family arrangements. The media might offer images of grandparents raising grandchildren. Legislation and social institutions such as schools, social service agencies, employers, and medical groups can begin recognizing and defining parenting based on who is providing primary care, rather than exclusively on who provided genetic material. With this research, I join the ranks of other kinship care researchers and scholars of reproduction, motherhood, and science studies who are bringing these questions to light in a productive manner.

REFERENCES

Alternative to dumping newborns: New law allows infants to be left at hospital, no questions asked. (2001, January 1). *San Francisco Examiner*, p. A1.

Bartholet, E. (1999). *Nobody's children: Abuse, neglect, foster drift, and the adoption alternative*. Boston: Beacon Press.

Burlingham-Brown, B. (1994). *"Why didn't she keep me?" Answers to the question every adopted child asks*. South Bend, IN: Langford Books.

Connolly, D. (2000a). *Homeless mothers: Face to face with women and poverty*. Minneapolis: University of Minnesota Press.

Connolly, D. (2000b). Mythical mothers and dichotomies of good and evil: Homeless mothers in the United States. In H. Ragoné & F. W. Twine (Eds.), *Ideologies and technologies of motherhood* (pp. 263-294). New York: Routledge Press.

Coontz, S. (1992). *The way we never were: American families and the nostalgia trap*. New York: Basic Books.

Cox, C. B. (Ed.). (2000). *To grandmother's house we go and stay: Perspectives on custodial grandparents*. New York: Springer Publishing Company.

Crosbie-Burnett, M. & Lewis, E. (1999). Use of African-American family structures and functioning to address the challenges of European-American post-divorce families. In S. Coontz, M. Parson, & G. Raley (Eds.), *American families: A multicultural reader* (pp. 455-469). New York: Routledge Press.

Crumbley, J. & Little, R. L. (Eds.). (1997). *Relatives raising children: An overview of kinship care*. Washington, DC: Child Welfare League of America Press.

Gailey, C. W. (2000). Ideologies of motherhood and kinship in U.S. adoption. In H. Ragoné & F. W. Twine (Eds.), *Ideologies and technologies of motherhood* (pp. 11-55). New York: Routledge Press.

Gleeson, J. P. & Hairston, C. F. (Eds.). (1999). *Kinship care: Improving practice through research*. Washington, DC: Child Welfare League of America Press.

Gordon, L. (1994). *Pitied but not entitled: Single mothers and the history of welfare.* New York: Free Press.

Hegar, R. L. & Scannapieco, M. (Eds.). (1999). *Kinship foster care: Policy practice and research.* New York: Oxford University Press.

Ladd-Taylor, M. & Umansky, L. (Eds.). (1998). *"Bad" mothers: The politics of blame in twentieth century America.* New York: New York University Press.

Murphy, S. & Rosenbaum, M. (1999). *Pregnant women on drugs: Combating stereotypes and stigma.* New Brunswick, NJ: Rutgers University Press.

Polakow, V. (1993). *Lives on the edge: Single mothers and their children in the other America.* Chicago: University of Chicago Press.

Ragoné, H. & Twine, F. W. (Eds.). (2000). *Ideologies and technologies of motherhood.* New York: Routledge Press.

Schneider, D. (1968). *American kinship: A cultural account.* Chicago: University of Chicago Press.

Sidel, R. (1992). *Women and children last: The plight of poor women in affluent America.* New York: Penguin Books.

Stack, C. (1974). *All our kin: Strategies for survival in a black community.* New York: Harper and Row.

Tsing, A. L. (1990). Monster stories: Women charged with perinatal endangerment. In F. Ginsburg & A. L. Tsing (Eds.), *Uncertain terms: Negotiating gender in American culture* (pp. 282-299). Boston: Beacon Press.

Chapter 9

Looking Promising:
Contradictions and Challenges
for Young Mothers in Care

Marilyn Callahan
Deborah Rutman
Susan Strega
Lena Dominelli

This chapter focuses on a unique and largely invisible group of mothers—young women in the care of government. These women have lived apart from their own parents for some or all of their lives. They now have children whom they may be mothering or who may have been removed from them on a temporary or permanent basis. The state serves as both their parent and their children's grandparent, often reluctantly and through an ever-changing number of surrogate family members including foster and group home parents and residents, staff in various community agencies, and social workers responsible for overseeing both their care and the protection of their children.

Although some research has focused on adolescent pregnancy and mothering (Allen & Bourke-Dowling, 1998; Appell, 1998; Flanagan, 1998; Gorlick, 1994; Horowitz, 1995; Hudson & Ineichen, 1991; Jacobs, 1994; Lawson & Rhode, 1993; Phoenix, 1991), only a few studies have addressed the particular situation and experiences of young women in government care (Horton, 1997; Mullins & McCluskey, 1999). The emerging literature on youth in care (Strega, 2000; Rutman, Strega, Callahan & Dominelli, 2002) has not focused particularly on those young people who are mothers.

Lone mothers are being increasingly demonized in popular and public policy discourse (Harris, 1997; Sidel, 1996). They are not only described as a serious financial burden on the state but their existence is cited as evidence of encroaching moral decay. Some mothers are more valued than others, and when the "wrong" women give birth, moral, psychological, and health concerns come to the fore (Phoenix, Woollett, & Lloyd, 1991). In this particular climate it is not surprising that government does not shine a light on its own "daughters" who are giving birth in surprising numbers[1] while in their teens (Martin, 1995, 1996).

We are a group of researchers with a keen interest in the lives of these young women, emerging in large part from our varied experiences in child welfare practice. One author began her social work practice as a child welfare worker and remembers clearly many young women in care who became pregnant while in foster care or who were taken into care because of early pregnancies. These young women may have remained in their foster homes for the duration of their pregnancies but were often sent away in later months to the church-based homes for unwed mothers documented in compelling fashion in the book *Gone to an Aunt's: Remembering Canada's Homes for Unwed Mothers* (Petrie, 1998). The policies and practices of the time encouraged social workers to remove infants from mothers at birth and place the children for adoption, expecting young women to resume their teen years as if these births had not occurred.

Another author of this chapter was a young woman taken into care at age eleven who did not get pregnant but remembers clearly her precarious life in foster care. At present, one author is working with youth in care for a research project and has heard many firsthand accounts of their lives. All of us have the experience of mothering in one form or another and bring these varied experiences to this research enterprise.

Precious little attention is given to what it means to be raised by the state. There is virtually no understanding of what it means to be a mother in these circumstances where grandparenting occurs only if mothering fails. This chapter examines the experiences of mothering in the context of these realities and proposes a theory to explain how some young women are constructed as worthy to be mothers and others are not.

THE RESEARCH METHODOLOGY

The researchers used a grounded theory method, an approach that begins with the lived experiences of the participants (Gilgun, 1994) and focuses on the social processes involved in that experience and the relationship between the individual and the social and political context in which she lives (Strauss & Corbin, 1990). In-depth interviews were carried out as guided conversations, and the transcripts were coded after completion by each member of the research team, looking for significant interactions or "what the participants anguish over the most" (Keddy, Sims, & Noerager Stern, 1996). Next, these open codes were clustered together in related processes. The researchers also engaged in memo writing, sampled the extensive literature on adolescent pregnancy and mothering/parenting, and shared preliminary theoretical findings with a participant focus group and an advisory committee composed of young mothers, social workers, policy analysts, and community workers.

The young women in our study included eleven participants living in urban and rural areas of southern Vancouver Island, British Columbia. They ranged in age from sixteen to twenty-four years and had been thirteen to eighteen years of age at the time of their first pregnancy. Three were Aboriginal. Eight of the women had their child(ren) living with them full-time at the time of the interview, although a few had their children removed from them at some point. Two of the women shared parenting with government agencies, caring for their children on a part-time basis, and one mother lived apart from her child who was in government care. Our intention as researchers was to interview participants who reflect the diversity of young women who have children while in care. As previously mentioned, we were unable to obtain a profile of this population. We also held four focus groups with First Nations workers, social workers responsible for young mothers in care, and other community workers. Finally, we conducted a policy review, tracing the history and development of those policies identified by young mothers as most influential on their lives, and noting policy gaps.

The agency responsible for caring for children and youth in British Columbia, Canada, where this study was undertaken, the Ministry for Child and Family Development (MCFD), is one of the largest government departments in the province and includes a wide range of social services. Although policymaking is centralized, services are delivered throughout the province primarily through social work staff situated in local offices. Many services to families are contracted out to local nonprofit and for-profit social service organizations, and much of the social worker's job involves developing and monitoring the work contracts of others. Social workers, however, receive delegation authority from the director of child welfare, the child's legal guardian, and act for the guardian in day-to-day decisions affecting the lives of children and youth in care. Young people are keenly aware of the power of their social workers vis-à-vis other helpers.

THE FINDINGS: LOOKING PROMISING

Elsewhere, we have reported that the experiences of young mothers in care could be conceptualized as "prevailing on the edge on my own" (Strega, Callahan, Rutman, & Dominelli, 2000; Callahan, Strega, Rutman, & Dominelli, 2003). The concept of "prevailing" contains within it a great deal of individual agency, of courage and sometimes triumph over highly adverse circumstances. It both encapsulates and goes beyond surviving. "On the edge," by contrast, signifies destabilizing and disempowering forces beyond the capacity of individual actions to address. These destabilizing forces sometimes emerged from the child welfare services themselves. The third concept, "on my own," reflects the ways that relationships between young women and others, while sometimes enriching, were often fragile, even with their own children. Again the policy and practice of child welfare contributed to this sense of being alone. In the intersection of these three concepts, we observed a dramatic and ever-present tension within the young women of being able to act powerfully and feeling powerless. We also observed the enormous emotional energy required to balance these tensions and to feel positive about oneself.

Upon completing this stage of the data analysis, we recognized that we had a rich description of the lives of young women, particularly their struggles to mother their children, but we were unable to explain what accounted for the differences in their experiences. Clearly some young women were "prevailing on the edge on their own" much better than others, according to their own assessments. Some were raising their children, although struggling; others had their children removed. Some had dreams while scrambling to manage day-to-day realities; others seemed overwhelmed by these realities. We needed some explanatory variables: a theory, grounded in the experiences of young mothers in care, that would explain the diversity in these experiences.

We returned to the data from the young women and from the focus groups of service providers to determine what might account for these variations. We were struck by the importance of the interactions between social workers and young women. What social workers thought about the different young women and how young women positioned themselves with their workers was key to understanding differences in experiences.

We determined that some young women looked promising to workers, with the potential to break the cycle of poverty and a tumultuous childhood and adolescence, and overcome the poor parenting the state had provided. They seemed able to raise themselves out of their working-class background and aspire to middle-class values and behaviors. These young women seemed deserving of the social worker's help and able to use what the social workers could offer (assistance with launching tasks, education, and child care). Most critically, being deserving meant being able to keep one's child—being deserving of motherhood.

LOOKING PROMISING:
WHAT YOUNG WOMEN THOUGHT

For young women, looking promising and breaking the cycle consisted of many interrelated processes that we have summarized into three main actions. Young women did not suggest that they had necessarily mastered these processes, nor did they make direct connections between these processes and success with social workers and others in the system. Rather, these were the challenges that they identified as being essential to their survival as young mothers in care.

Triumphing over a Truncated and Harrowing Childhood

Young women were proud of their accomplishments in living through what could hardly be termed a childhood. Many had left home at an early age, sometimes as young as three years, and they had learned to live in the precarious and unloving circumstances of state care. Some had simply left home for the streets and had survived the dangers of drugs, prostitution, and homelessness.

I'm only eighteen, but I feel like I'm forty-five years old.

Being with my mother, I grew up really quickly. I had to look after her and cook for her and all her party animal friends that came over.

As children and youths, they needed to learn how to deal with social workers, foster parents, and other helpers and to be, we argue, raised by policy rather than parents.

I grew up with no control over what MCFD wanted or expected of me. I wasn't given the chance to say, "Yeah, I would like to live in a Native home."— I was never raised on choices. I was raised on, "You are doing this, and this is the way it has to be."

Among the challenges was learning how to develop and then lose relationships that matter. There was a strong message about the importance overall of the relationship with social workers, seen as stand-in parents with the power to make significant changes in their lives.

Although these young women had few opportunities to experience childhood as it is traditionally conceived, they tended to minimize these losses when speaking to others, particularly social workers, lest they appear ill prepared for adulthood and mothering. Thus, they were particularly conscious of not appearing to be typical teens, crazy about boys and with no eye to the future. Most talked about having dreams and aspirations that ensured they would be financially and personally independent.

Yeah, I'm a single parent. I was a teenage mom—okay, sure. But I'm not going to sit on welfare for the rest of my life. I'm not going to have my kids apprehended from me. I'm not going to screw the Ministry.

Demonstrating Good Mothering Under Adversity

Having a child at an early age was a turning point for all the young women. They remarked consistently that pregnancy and birth had saved them or could have saved them from a destructive, even fatal, set of circumstances and made them want to live for someone else's sake.

I had opportunities to get off the streets, but because being on the streets was such an easy life to live, I chose that. But becoming pregnant, it was like, "Well, now I have to think of two people." But [my daughter's] a part of me. So really, if I was maybe thinking of one person [myself], she just smartened me up and got me off [the streets].

Pregnancy occurred at a young age for all of these women, but most had engaged in behavior well beyond their years at all stages of their lives, such as taking care of their own parents and siblings, moving from residence to residence while in care, and living on their own on the streets. In some ways, they were much older than their years, making pregnancy and motherhood less surprising than for teens their age who had led more protected lives.

Young women were very conscious about what others thought was good mothering, even though most of them had never experienced such mothering themselves. They identified tasks such as providing for their children, keeping to a routine, staying out of the party scene, and providing their children with love and guidance. These tasks appear similar to what other mothers might say. These young women in government care, however, had very high expectations of themselves and were determined to accomplish these tasks even without adequate financial resources and the support of an extended and consistent family. Most did not have stable partners to share parenting. They attempted to create or re-create family by connecting with their own parents and siblings and the families of their boyfriends and by appealing to social workers and others who could offer resources.

When [my daughter] comes home, I'm going to be a different person than when she left. I'll be someone she looks forward to coming home to, and not saying, "Oh, my mom's mad. I don't want to go there right now."

I learned how to cook with a screaming kid, clean with a screaming kid, take a shower with a screaming kid. [The staff at the home for adolescent mothers] teach you a lot of responsibility.

Part of being a good mother was scrounging for resources from many quarters. To do so, young women needed to gain knowledge of a large number of systems and present themselves appropriately to these resources. Much of their conversation focused on a detailed inventory of government and community resources, eligibility criteria, and the arbitrary nature in which they were deployed by social workers. Among their challenges was learning how to position themselves as in need and yet competent enough to continue to care for their children. In British Columbia, this is particularly challenging, because parents can receive support services from government only if their children are at risk. Mothers fear the at-risk label, worrying that it could be used against them in future child protection investigations.

Keeping or Regaining Custody of My Child

All the young women spoke fervently about the need to keep their own children out of government care. The fear of losing a child to care and the struggles to avoid being investigated permeated their talk.

> That's why, well, like, from, I, you know when you get pregnant. So you just feel different. And from that point I stopped doing drugs, I stopped smoking, and I stopped drinking. I stopped everything. And I've, gotten drunk twice since he's been born. And I won't even do that anymore. Because I guess I just, that would be my worst fear. If somebody tried to take him away. And, it's just been an awful fear in the back of my mind.

To lose a child to state care, as they had been lost, was a truly significant sign of failure, even though some acknowledged that they were not able to care for their children at some stages of their lives or even at present. One young woman described a friend's experience when her child was removed by the state:

> I've supported a friend of mine who had to go through that. And it was just horrendous. 'Cause they have the right to get a hearing for that really quick. I think it's within twenty-four or forty-eight hours or something like that. But then it keeps getting remanded and remanded and remanded. So you know, nothing gets settled really quick, even though they have the right to a hearing real quick. And it's just horrible. And I've gone through that with women as far back as five years ago. And it still affects her children to this day. These kids still can't go for sleepovers at friends' houses anymore without having to call their mom and say, "I want to come home. I want to come home. I don't want to stay here anymore."

They felt that the eyes of the state and community were on them at all times: while riding the bus, trying to shop, in the housing projects, at family gatherings, when they went to the physician and the welfare office, and when their social workers came to visit. They knew that there were files on them from their childhoods and that their youthful behavior was part and parcel of how social workers judged them now as mothers. They talked about the social workers' use of risk assessments and feared the application of these assessments to themselves.

Part of the process of keeping their children out of care involved demonstrating that they were different. Young women frequently distanced themselves from others in the same boat, lest they be tarnished with the stereotypes of lone mothers. Young women constantly remarked that they were different from other young women of the same age and other lone mothers. They were also determined to be different from their own mothers.

> Do I want to live like my mother and be the way my mother was to my child, or am I going to stop that cycle and be somebody different?

At the same time, they often needed to reconnect with friends and their family to assist with their own mothering tasks.

LOOKING PROMISING: WHAT SOCIAL WORKERS THOUGHT

Not surprisingly, busy social workers with large caseloads viewed the challenges facing young mothers and themselves somewhat differently. These findings have been reported in depth but are summarized here (Rutman et al., 2002). Although social workers did not explicitly identify the following three processes as important in surviving the experience of being young mothers in care, these findings emerged from their talk.

Avoiding Motherhood in Care

> She got pregnant in a foster home—so yeah, I was kind of saddened by that. 'Cause I thought that maybe she was, I was feeling hopeful for her. Now I'm not feeling quite so hopeful anymore for her.

And this one girl, I was really happy or heartened that she would say to me and her foster mother, after years of chaotic abusive history, that she didn't want to repeat the cycle. That she wanted to be—she wanted to get on with her life. She wanted to be more of a success than her peers. She wanted to take the example of what's happened to her and break the cycle. . . . And then she went and got pregnant. *And of course the child was apprehended and now she's pregnant again.* [emphasis added]

Ideally, social workers hoped that young woman would not get pregnant in the first place because, for workers, pregnancy provided confirmation that a young woman was repeating the cycle. To get pregnant so young seemed to confirm workers' stereotypes of certain classes and races of women; indeed, these young women were behaving much like their own mothers—mothers who had lost their children to care. Workers feared that young women raised in care would be unable to mother because of the inadequacies of the state parenting that they experienced. Pregnancy was perceived as both worker failure and failure on the part of the young women to break the cycle. As one worker stated:

Our job is to see that they don't get pregnant if we can, which is impossible.

Thus while the young women were trying to break the cycle by demonstrating their mothering capacities, their workers viewed them as perpetuating it through these activities.

Demonstrating Good Mother Behavior

Workers accepted that those who did become mothers could nonetheless break the cycle if they proved themselves capable of good mothering. Both workers and young women agreed that being a good mother consisted of understanding the essential ingredients of mothering and demonstrating behaviors such as producing clean houses, well-behaved children on routines, and so forth. As one worker stated:

And I went to her house one time to do a CPOC [a protection investigation] and she had that place so organized and so immaculate. And I thought, wow, this girl really is, this young woman is really taking being a parent seriously.

Both groups shared the belief that the only way to break the cycle was by providing different (adequate) mothering than the young women themselves received. Workers acknowledged their belief that it was very difficult for young women to be good mothers, in spite of the young women's determination. While young women were trying to prove their abilities, workers worried that the cycle was being repeated in the lives of the children.

Workers acknowledged the scrutiny that young mothers had mentioned:

> They'll certainly be under much more scrutiny. They're under much more scrutiny than someone who's not, that's not in the system. Because you have that contact. We've all got references and flags, etc., because when you see something going down, it may you know, it's going to be a different standard than someone who's not come to the attention of the Ministry.

They believed that if they did not ensure sufficient surveillance over the young women, their own jobs and professional futures were at risk. Workers were also aware that they could not really offer young mothers what they needed and parceled out services to those who they thought could use them best. Some workers were aware of this classing process that rewarded those most likely to fit middle-class norms.

> We're a middle-class organization and we have middle-class values that we're trying to impose on clients who may or may not have middle-class values.

> We do have middle-class values. I can remember one of my clients who was seventeen and wanted to have a baby, and the psychologist said, "Well, you know, if this was in her own people's lives she would have had two or three by now." Just 'cause you think education is important—which I got to admit is my bias. You know—it would be normal for her but our system says: you go through in a middle-class way, and you do this and this and this. And a lot of our clients are not on board with that.

Although many workers held strong values and beliefs regarding the inevitability of the cycle of poor parenting and children's entry into care, they also fundamentally understood the relationship between a young mother's poverty and the likelihood of her surveillance by the child protection arm of the Ministry:

Like they really believe, it's like they honestly, I don't know of any one of the kids that I've worked with, or youth I've worked with, who didn't really believe that they were going to break the chain. That they were going to treat their child differently than they were. But they forget that at two o'clock in the morning the baby wakes up and needs changing his diapers. And if you don't have the money for diapers or don't have diapers, what do you do? Or you don't have food in the fridge to feed it.

Indeed, many workers spoke passionately about the state's inadequate funding for young mothers in care. Workers knew that it was almost impossible to find adequate housing given current housing allowances. Workers also knew that without safe, decent housing young mothers would be subjected to the Ministry's scrutiny and possible child protection investigation. Thus, legislated poverty set up young mothers for failure, and workers, as parents/guardians, were embarrassed and often outraged to be complicit actors in this state-sanctioned negligence.

I'm appalled that we allow our children in care to live under the poverty line. I think that the government is just disgusting, and it's just appalling to me that these people who we're supposed to be guardians of, we're allowing to live in poverty and deprivation. And it's been going on for the twenty years that I've been working in this Ministry. And it's sad. It's absolutely sad.

You know, when I look at our kids, most of their money goes into having a decent place to live, and if you don't have a decent place to live then your kid comes to our attention.

Being a Good Daughter

Workers' hopes for young women were similar to those they might have for any young woman, including daughters: a good education, a decent-paying job, an ability to live independently and have strong friendships and support, a stable partner, a home, and healthy children. To reach these goals, workers thought that it was particularly important that young women have other aspirations and abilities besides mothering. Mothering consumed much of the energies of young women, but workers believed that young women who continued in school, had plans to graduate, attended parenting classes, and got involved in activities to better themselves were those with promise. The class and cultural basis for these expectations was rarely explored.

First Nations women, in particular, struggled to understand these norms and had difficulty appearing to meet them.

Moreover, workers expected more from these young mothers than they would from their own daughters. They knew that after young women were discharged from care at nineteen years of age, they would have very little in the way of benefits and support. They tried to prepare them for independence at age nineteen, an expectation that is not placed on young people not in care. Indeed, middle-class youths are expected to remain dependent on their parents for several years beyond. Canadian provincial and federal government programs increasingly expect parental support for postsecondary education, supplementary income, and other forms of material support for those beginning work and other launching tasks of young adulthood.

LOOKING PROMISING: A BEGINNING THEORY

Our study reflects the experiences of young women who, in the main, wish to be hands-on mothers and their social workers who doubt their capacity to do so. It points to several taken-for-granted assumptions that come between the aspirations of these young women and those of their social workers. Although these assumptions seem to live beneath the terrain of professional and public thinking, they exert powerful influences. Our study underscored the particular influence of one of these assumptions, breaking the cycle.

Young mothers were deeply committed to breaking the cycle. For them, the cycle consisted of being mired in a rootless life involving the street scene, possibly drugs and prostitution, frequent AWOL periods from foster and group homes, and a lack of stability or long-term prospects. Although they did not use the term delinquent, they clearly felt on the fringes of young offender or child welfare law and policies. They were intent on breaking the delinquent cycle—their assumption being that young women in trouble grow up to be women with more serious troubles.

Young mothers also worried about breaking another cycle: those children who were poorly mothered will grow up to be poor mothers. All felt particularly passionate about breaking this cycle, although examples of their own neglect and abuse by their parents and surrogate parents were fresh in their minds, and the removal of some of their children confirmed that it was going to be very challenging to accomplish this.

Not surprisingly, they became pregnant at young ages. From their perspective, pregnancy gave them a chance to break both of these cycles: to leave the streets or their unsettled lives in care, and to demonstrate their capacities as mothers.

Our respondents also expressed the uncomfortable feeling that they had already been discarded by professionals because, by becoming teenagers and then mothers, they were already too old to be changed. Although they felt that they received more attention from social workers when they became pregnant, the attention seemed to focus on their unborn children who had the potential to break the cycle.

Social workers were also concerned about breaking the cycle, but they focused more on the cycle of dependency. Those who grow up dependent upon government care will likely remain on government programs as adults. In other words, young girls in foster care will become welfare mothers. Social workers' jobs were to help young women become independent from the government services that were their surrogate families and go it alone as adults.

As workers endure many discouraging outcomes, difficult working conditions, and high caseloads, they are attracted to those young women who appear to be breaking the cycle. Looking promising is a stance that gains support and resources from beleaguered helping systems; workers triage those cases that they think have the most chance of success. Young women who, in the workers' words, "seem to be making it" against these odds by not getting pregnant or by keeping their children and getting educated, or by getting out on their own, rekindled workers' hopes that success was possible. Those most likely to appear to be making it are articulate white women who already look the part and who may have figured out how the system works. By looking promising, young women attract the approval and at least some modest resources required to meet or appear to meet their almost overwhelming tasks. A self-fulfilling prophecy is at work. For young women, their positive relationship with a social worker was particularly important in this process.

Those who are unlikely to look promising shared certain characteristics: they looked poor, were more likely to be First Nations, and had demonstrated difficulty both in mothering and in becoming independent under highly adverse conditions. As a result, they did not attract the necessary relationships and resources to change this impression, and, if their mothering were investigated and/or a child removed, they were even less likely to be able to reposition themselves as promising.

Our theory requires testing but fits with our sample and has resonance with young mothers and social workers who attended a forum at which we presented our findings (Rutman, Hubberstey, Barlow, Alusik, & Brown, 2001). Moreover, aspects of our theory are supported by other research. Studies document that young women struggling to overcome daunting problems in adolescence view motherhood as a way of getting a grip on their lives (Flanagan, 1998; Lawson & Rhode, 1993).

Holland's (2000) study of the verbal interactions between investigating social workers and parents supports our assertion that how a mother presents herself to the worker is important. Holland concluded that those parents who were described by the social worker as working well within the assessment relationship were also described as articulate, providing plausible explanations for their behavior, and as cooperative and motivated to accept and conform to social workers' expectations. Furthermore, family reunification was most likely in these cases. Those identified as "passive parents" were perceived by workers to be inarticulate, inconsistent, and lacking appropriate emotional responses. Griffiths's (1995) study of conversations between mothers and teachers lends further support to the importance of appearing to be a middle-class mother in order to gain benefits for children. Those mothers able to converse in the child development discourse and their children were regarded more favorably by elementary school teachers than those who could not, usually poor women and/or women of color.

MAINTAINING THE CYCLE: POLICY OBSERVATIONS

Our analysis of policy affecting young women and their workers (Strega, Callahan, Rutman, & Dominelli, 2002) indicates that policy works against young women's efforts to break the cycle of poor mothering and state care for their children, and workers' efforts to break the cycle of state dependence. We suggest that belief in the in-

evitability of the cycle actually ensures that these cycles will continue, providing them with further credibility and influence. Although it is beyond the scope of this chapter to examine policies in
depth, a few require particular mention.

For young women to demonstrate that they have risen above a trau-
matic and truncated childhood is not easy, given the policies that have
shaped and continue to shape the parenting that they have been offered. Although workers' assessments of mothers' abilities emphasize the need for mothers to provide stable, long-term, and caring relationships to their children, the state does not hold itself to this same
standard. State parenting is precarious, and the issue of who is really
doing the parenting is obscured. It is organized so that the core feature
of parenting, that is, long-term caring relationships between the surrogate parent (the social worker) and the child, becomes highly unlikely. In British Columbia, intake and investigation is performed by
one team, protective family services are provided by another, and
guardianship services, which support those in care, are handled by a
third group. The demanding and frustrating nature of child welfare
work continues to contribute to turnover among workers that is
higher than in other fields. In addition, foster parents and group home
staff struggle with inadequate remuneration and support, often leading them to quit.

Other policies result in children experiencing frequent moves.
Care provided in foster families and group homes is frequently cate-
gorized according to levels of children's behavior, with the most
compensation awarded to caregivers who take children deemed most
problematic. As children improve, they are moved to another re-
source. Services for children and foster parents are contracted out to
nonprofit and for-profit organizations, usually to the lowest bidder
and often on an annual basis, resulting in frequent personnel changes.
One young woman sums up the situation clearly.

> Because relationships with people when you are in care keep changing.
> I mean group homes. Group homes keep changing. You keep getting
> bounced and bounced around and around. And then within that group
> home, there is youth that are coming in and out, and in and out, and in and
> out. And there is staff that is coming in and out, in and out, in and out. Then
> your social workers, like, come and go and come and go and go and go. And
> it's just, there is nothing consistent or stable. And I think that is the hardest
> thing for me, when I made that transition out of government care, was I con-
> tinued that, and I didn't know what stability or any of that really was.

Some jurisdictions have developed policies to help young people move out of care and to continue support to them beyond the age of eighteen or nineteen years; however, these policies are recent, over-subscribed, often encourage early employment in low-wage jobs, and pay little if any attention to parenting responsibilities. Those young people who move out of care onto welfare benefits will receive increasingly inadequate and insecure benefits.

Policies supporting young women to provide adequate care to their children and to deal with the stigma and surveillance that they experience are similarly counterproductive. Although the state has legal responsibility for a young woman in its care, it assumes no grand-parenting responsibilities for the child she bears. Some provisions may be made for her child on a discretionary basis, but resources such as day care or respite care will be provided only if the child is assessed as being at risk or becomes a ward of government, the very event that young women are trying to avoid. This policy direction, of providing supportive parenting services only for those children deemed to be at risk as measured on risk-assessment instruments, is a feature of British Columbia's child welfare policy and is emerging in other Canadian provinces. High-profile child neglect and abuse scandals have led governments to introduce risk-assessment instruments as concrete evidence of their action to prevent such tragedies. However, as several researchers have demonstrated, little if any relationship exists between scores on risk-assessment instruments and the likelihood that a child will be abused or neglected in the future (English & Pecora, 1994; Houston & Griffiths, 2000; Parton, 1998). Furthermore, many of the items on the risk-assessment form penalize young women from the beginning: their young age, single status, possible or previous involvement with drugs and alcohol, their inadequate income, the fact that they are in care, their inadequate housing, and so on.

A final feature of policies affecting young mothers in care is the lack of clear and coherent policy direction regarding their situations. Young mothers do not have a statutory right to support services and educational or income programs. They may be eligible for some or all of these programs, depending upon many variables, including assessment by their social workers. This policy vacuum may explain, in part, the individual and discretionary approach toward young women described by the workers in our research. Workers cobble together a policy response to the situation of wards and their children, using other policies at their discretion. Mothers feel the ambiguities of policy and are constantly trying to learn the latest policy developments, find out what happened to others in their situation, and position themselves favorably with their workers. Their preoccupation with looking promising, and thus deserving, is a congruent response to a policy vacuum that provides little direction for workers aside from insisting on fiscal and administrative imperatives.

CONTRADICTIONS AND OBSTACLES IN BREAKING THE CYCLE

The fundamental notion that delinquency, neglect, abuse, and dependency will be transmitted from one generation to the next unless some kind of external intervening force is applied has framed thinking in child welfare since its formal inception at the turn of the century. Neglected children and some needy mothers were among the few groups characterized as deserving in early social policy development. As was true in other jurisdictions in Canada, initial efforts in British Columbia focused on saving children from the immorality and ineptness of their parents.[2] In support of early child welfare legislation in British Columbia in 1901, a Supreme Court justice offered this embryonic cycle theory, which has since his time come to be understood as truth:

> [T]he children of drunken and immoral parents should have protection by law so as to enable them to grow up to live a useful life and not by force of their surroundings becoming untruthful, unclean and immoral and add to the pauper and criminal class of the community. (Singleton cited in Callahan & Wharf, 1982, p. 7)

In effect, child welfare is founded on a simple proposition: Removing children from inadequate parents (which, in practice, is usually the inadequate care offered by mothers) and introducing them to the lives of the middle class will result in these same children embracing middle-class values of discipline and independence. Child welfare is and has been a clear and failed attempt to assimilate the lower classes into the middle, and the nonwhite into the white on a case-by-case basis and to deny the strong relationship between structural inequalities related to class, race, and gender and what has been adjudged to be bad parenting (Swift, 1995, 1997; Wharf, 1993).

Breaking the cycle has gained additional credibility in child welfare through professional discourses founded upon both traditional and progressive theories about child and family development. The notion that children will absorb the psychological imperfections of their parents unless wise and disciplined professional intervention occurs is a foundation of social science research and professional education. From Freudian notions of repressed Oedipal functioning to Bowlby's attachment theory and the present focus on transmission of sexual abuse and family violence through generations, there is an unwavering commitment to the necessity of breaking the cycle.

With some exceptions, these ideological and professional discourses rest on the assumption that parental failures stem from individual pathology rather than social conditions or structural inequalities. They also fit with a fundamental assumption of Western European thinking concerning the value of progress, defined as being different from and thus better than the previous generation.

Our study suggests that young women who believe that they can break the cycle by demonstrating their capacity to be good mothers face a number of significant contradictions and obstacles:

1. Young women who become mothers in their teens disappoint their social workers who believe that they are continuing the cycle of youthful and inadequate parenting and long-term dependency on welfare.
2. Young women must demonstrate their capacity to earn an independent living and be an adequate mother, while lacking the resources to do either.
3. Young women must be prepared for independent living by age nineteen, including caring for a child, even though they have had few supports to do so. By contrast, most young people without children and not in government care rely upon their families for many years past their nineteenth birthday.
4. Young women who are in care have likely experienced inadequate parenting, which is considered a risk factor when social workers examine young mothers' care of their own children. However, the state itself frequently provided the inadequate parenting for these young women and now blames them for its own inadequacies.

5. Young women believe that being a good mother requires having emotional and financial support, but because they are in care, it is hard for them to connect to their families for such support or to social workers who are frequently constrained from providing all necessary support.
6. Young women wanting to gain support for mothering must indicate that the safety and well-being of their children will be at risk unless support is given. However, by agreeing to such a position, they put themselves and their children at risk for further child protection investigations.
7. Young women in care know that their files contain damaging information about them as children and teenagers, and such files can be used to judge their suitability for mothering, even if they have made changes in their lives since becoming mothers.
8. Young women know that their children will be provided with more benefits if they relinquish custody of them, since social workers can provide financial support for substitute parents to care for children but cannot do the same for birth mothers.
9. Young women who understand that middle-class values and ways of talking will impress social workers are usually least in need of assistance and yet most likely to get it. Those who are hostile, silent, not white, or not aspiring to middle-class goals will look least promising and are less likely to receive the help they badly need.
10. Social workers know that maintaining surveillance over young mothers is a self-defeating activity, as it is difficult to do and undermines young mothers' confidence. However, if social workers do not maintain surveillance, they risk their own jobs should something go wrong.
11. Young women appreciate that they have been branded as someone who needs to break the cycle because they have spent some or all of their childhood and youth in government care. They know that they must prove themselves yet feel stigmatized and marginalized. Close relationships providing acceptance, mentoring, and consistency—the key ingredients required to help them overcome their challenges—are rarely possible with government workers, given the organization of government work.

12. Young women believe that they already may be too old to look like promising people who will break the cycle and that the attention they need is directed toward their very young children.

Young women and their social workers feel the impact of these contradictions:

We don't go in and put someone into a home to help them parent better. We take the kids out and give them to someone who is supposedly a better parent. One of the things the system doesn't recognize, because there is such a cut [in resources], is that some of the parenting was good and some of it wasn't so good. But we don't fix families, we break them apart. [social worker]

What I feel is not right is when young moms try as hard as they can, they jump through all the hoops and run that extra mile, and they do not say "good job" or "nice try." We do not get any recognition for what we are doing. Somehow they still make us feel we are not doing anything right and that we are not going to be good moms. How are we supposed to be doing good when we keep on being put down, and they make it seem we cannot do anything right or good? I wish the Ministry would work for us instead of against us. [young mother]

That young women have difficulty mothering their children under these circumstances should come as no surprise. The explanation that they are unable to break the cycle is simply unacceptable and denies the complicity of public policy and professional practice in creating cycles that are impossible to break.

We have suggestions for breaking the cycle. At present, provincial government policy aimed at breaking the cycle involves tightening eligibility for welfare for lone mothers and using risk-management approaches to determine child neglect and abuse. These policies have had predictable results: increasing numbers of children entering state care and a reduction in resources to mothers to reclaim their children. Instead we suggest policies and practices that (1) are based on expressed need rather than potential of risk; (2) consider the experiences of children in their own homes and in state care when choosing the least detrimental alternative for mother and child (Arad & Wozner, 2001); and (3) are grounded in group and community approaches to child welfare (Wharf, 2002). These approaches have the potential for breaking cyclical thinking and responding to the issues of mothers and their children.

Finally, our study raises questions about how the importance of appearing to be a white, middle-class mother assumes more value than the actual caregiving that may be occurring in any particular situation. There are entrenched beliefs that those who are too "ethnic," or too young or too poor or too quiet or too hostile to workers simply cannot be giving the proper care to their children. Neither the definition of proper care nor the potential for prejudicial judgments are questioned. It is here in the world of white middle-class policy-making and professional practice where real change must occur.

NOTES

1. In spite of requests to the provincial ministry in charge of child welfare (British Columbia Ministry for Child and Family Development), we were unable to obtain a profile of young mothers in care, including their numbers. Ministry officials stated that they did not keep such data and that they were surprised that they did not, as they had the impression that pregnancy was a common occurrence among their wards. Polit, Morton, & Corette (1987) conclude that youth in foster care in the United States are twice as likely as their peers not in care to have had sexual intercourse; are less likely to be informed about human sexuality and birth control; are less likely to have used contraceptives during first intercourse or their most recent intercourse; are less likely to have obtained contraceptives at a family planning clinic; and are twice as likely to have been pregnant.

2. See Adamoski in Chapter 7 for a discussion of lone mothers and child rescue practices in Canada in the early twentieth century.

REFERENCES

Allen, I. & Bourke-Dowling, S., with Rolfe, H. (1998). *Teenage mothers: Decisions and outcomes.* London: Policy Studies Institute.

Appell, A. (1998). On fixing "bad" mothers and saving their children. In M. Ladd-Taylor & L. Umansky (Eds.), *"Bad" mothers: The politics of blame in twentieth-century America* (pp. 356-380). New York: University Press.

Arad, B. D. & Wozner, Y. (2001). The least detrimental alternative: Deciding whether to remove children at risk from their homes. *International Social Work* 44(2), 229-239.

Callahan, M., Strega, S., Rutman, D., & Dominelli, L. (2003). Undeserving mothers: Lived experience of young mothers in/from government care. In K. Kufeldt & B. McKenzie (Eds.), *Issues in Canadian child welfare* (pp. 249-260). Waterloo, ON: Wilfrid Laurier University Press.

Callahan, M. & Wharf, B. (1982). *Demystifying the policy process: A case study of the development of child welfare in B.C.* Victoria: Minuteman Press.

English, D. & Pecora, P. (1994). Risk assessment as a practice method in child protective services. *Child Welfare 73*(5), 451-473.

Flanagan, P. (1998). Teen mothers: Countering the myths of dysfunction and developmental disruption. In C. Coll, J. Surrey, & K. Weingarten (Eds.), *Mothering against the odds: Diverse voices of contemporary mothers* (pp. 238-254). New York: Guilford Press.

Gilgun, J. (1994). Hand into glove: The grounded theory approach and social work practice research. In E. Sherman & W. Reid (Eds.), *Qualitative research in social work* (pp. 115-125). New York: Columbia University Press.

Gorlick, C. (1994). Listening to low income children and single mothers: Policy implications related to child welfare. Paper presented at the National Research and Policy Symposium on Child Welfare, May 10-14, Kananaskis, AB.

Griffiths, A. (1995). Mothering, schooling and children's development. In M. Campbell & A. Manicom (Eds.), *Knowledge, experience and ruling relations* (pp. 108-121). Toronto: University of Toronto Press.

Harris, K. (1997). *Teen mothers and the revolving welfare door.* Philadelphia: Temple University Press.

Holland, S. (2000). The assessment relationship: Interactions between social workers and parents in child protection assessments. *British Journal of Social Work 30,* 149-163.

Horowitz, R. (1995). *Teen mothers: Citizens or dependents?* Chicago: University of Chicago Press.

Horton, J. (1997). Adolescent pregnancy and young women in care. *Canada's Children/Les Enfants du Canada 4*(2), 35-36.

Houston, S. & Griffiths, H. (2000). Reflections on risk in child protection: Is it time for a shift in paradigms? *Child and Family Social Work, 5*(1), 1-10.

Hudson, F. & Ineichen, B. (1991). *Taking it lying down: Sexuality and teenage motherhood.* London: MacMillan.

Jacobs, J. (1994). Gender, face, class and the trend toward early motherhood. *Journal of Contemporary Ethnography, 22*(4), 442-462.

Keddy, B., Sims, S., & Noerager Stern, P. (1996). Grounded theory as feminist research methodology. *Journal of Advanced Nursing, 23,* 446-453.

Lawson, A. & Rhode, D. (1993). *The politics of pregnancy: Adolescent sexuality and public policy.* New Haven, CT: Yale University Press.

Martin, F. (1995). Tales of transition: Gender differences in youth leaving care. *Canada's Children/Les Enfants du Canada, 2*(3), 21-24.

Martin, F. (1996). Tales of transition: Leaving public care. In B. Galaway & J. Hudson (Eds.), *Youth in transition: Perspectives on research and policy* (pp. 99-106). Toronto: Thompson.

Mullins, A. & McCluskey, J. (1999). *Teenage mothers speak for themselves.* London: Public Policy Unit.

Parton, N. (1998). Risk, advanced liberalism and child welfare: The need to rediscover uncertainty and ambiguity. *British Journal of Social Work, 28,* 5-27.

Petrie, A. (1998). *Gone to an aunt's: Remembering Canada's homes for unwed mothers*. Toronto: McClelland and Stewart.

Phoenix, A. (1991). Motherhood: Social construction, politics and psychology. In A. Phoenix, A. Woollett, & E. Lloyd (Eds.), *Motherhood: Meanings, practices and ideologies* (pp. 13-27). London: Sage.

Phoenix, A., Woollett, A., & Lloyd, E. (1991). *Motherhood: Meanings, practices and ideologies*. London: Sage.

Polit, D., Morton, T., & Corette, M. W. (1987). Sex, contraception and pregnancy among adolescents in foster care. *Family Planning Perspectives, 19*(1), 18-23.

Rutman, D., Hubberstey, C., Barlow, A., Alusik, D., & Brown, E. (2001). Supporting young people's transition from care. *Canada's Children/Les Enfants du Canada, 8*(3), 27-31.

Rutman, D., Strega, S., Callahan, M., & Dominelli, L. (2002). "Undeserving" mothers? Practitioners experience working with young mothers in/from care. *Child and Family Social Work, 7*(3), 149-159.

Sidel, R. (1996). *Keeping women and children last*. New York: Penguin Books.

Strauss, A. & Corbin, J. (1990). *Basics of qualitative research*. Newbury Park, CA: Sage.

Strega, S. (2000). Efforts at empowering youth: Youth-in-care and the youth-in-care networks in Ontario and Canada. In M. Callahan, S. Hessle, & S. Strega (Eds.), *Valuing the field: Child welfare in an international context* (pp. 4-22). Aldershot, UK: Ashgate Press.

Strega, S., Callahan, M., Rutman, D., & Dominelli, L. (2000). Undeserving mothers: Lived experiences of young mothers in/from government care. Joint Conference of the International Federation of Social Workers and the International Association of Schools of Social Work, Montreal, QB, August.

Strega, S., Callahan, M., Rutman, D., & Dominelli, L. (2002). "Bad" daughters who grow up to be "bad" mothers: A historical review of policies affecting young mothers who give birth in care. [Unpublished paper.] Victoria: University of Victoria.

Swift, K. (1995). *Manufacturing "bad mothers": A critical perspective on child neglect*. Toronto: University of Toronto Press.

Swift, K. (1997). Canada: Trends and issues in child welfare. In N. Gilbert (Ed.), *Combating child abuse: International perspectives and trends* (pp. 38-71). New York: Oxford University Press.

Wharf, B. (1993). *Rethinking child welfare*. Toronto: McClelland and Stewart.

Wharf, B. (2002). *Community approaches to child welfare*. Peterborough, ON: Broadview Press.

PART III:
COMBINING SITUATED KNOWLEDGES
OF MATERNAL ABSENCE

Chapter 10

Leaving to Grow/ Inspiration to Grow/ Leaving Inspiration

Gill Wright Miller

By definition, choreographers are mothers without children. Our creative offspring are notoriously spontaneous and ephemeral. To name dances is to refer to them only in the abstract, not so much in memory as in illusion; they exist only in the examples of performance, and in that sense we are always without them. Choreographers themselves make strong claims that the evidence of a dance is available only in its presence, as there is no tangibility to grasp, hold, or revere, and little kinesthetic satisfaction in the translation—photos, videos, or film. Only a distant record of something that once existed, some nonexperiential document (a program, a score, a video) or an experiential nondocument (a movement memory, an observational memory, a leftover injury) can stand in as confirmation that any creating occurred. Writers have published essays. Sculptors have commissioned statues. Painters have canvases. Choreographers have no tangible evidence that can be leaned carefully against a wall or slapped down on someone's desk to be still and await its evaluation: we are, indeed, mothers living without children.

I knew I had lived my whole professional life as a mother without children. And yet, as a biological mother of four, none of my friends or colleagues would ever have placed me in that category. This chapter serves as an exploration of that terrain: the margins where mothers are not mothering.

PROLOGUE

In spite of the professional résumé I can put together, my identity is bound up entirely by a deep and layered need to be successful as a mother. In my early twenties, I ranked having children far above developing myself as an artist. In my thirties, while chairing a blossoming, fast-paced dance department, I conceived of myself as first and foremost a mother by day, then a professor and administrator by night. In my forties, when I reflected on what I had accomplished, what I valued, what I yearned for, it was always an idealized relationship with my children. They inspired me, made me feel whole. What I failed to consider was the cultural coercion involved in striving to be valued as a daily on-site mother in the midst of the hour-by-hour work/home struggle. I had misunderstood what it means for a mother to be mothering.

My busy life as an academic was the epitome of multitasking, running from a first-grade play to concert performances, from a parent-teacher conference to chairs' meetings, from a high school tennis match to classes I was teaching. I baked cupcakes and graded papers into the wee hours of the night, throwing in laundry along the way. My sense of myself was that I was always behind, routinely gasping for breath. Artist friends from my late teens and early twenties had hopped on a different train long ago and were far away from me now. Suburban housewife friends were keeping up with school levies and village development in order to make the community better for all of our children. Professional colleagues were completing publishing projects that I only dreamed about. I found myself swimming in the currents of disappointment and frustration, even though I knew unequivocally that my children were the most intriguing art works I had spent a lifetime creating, shaping, and setting free to perform.

From time to time, however, occasional shifts occur in the phrasing of our lives. In these special suspended plateaus, revealed to us is simultaneously both past and present. Near my fortieth birthday, I reached for one of those plateaus by considering both the past twenty years and the next twenty years. In a conversation with my husband, I recounted for him the landmarks we had been taught to strive for: we had married, bought a home, had children, and made partner at the law firm and tenure at the university. The kinds of life events young adults with our backgrounds were supposed to want had been, miraculously, accomplished. We were approaching a pause.

What, I asked, did the next twenty years hold? What would be our panorama in this next phase, the score of years between creating ourselves and retiring? How do we provide for and parent adult children? What is our appropriate role? I felt the complex project I had been shepherding was drawing to completion and I had not yet identified the next challenge. I felt empty, directionless. Like a person who has just devoured a bag of potato chips, I was stuffed from the number of tasks that I accomplished each day but still hungry for sustenance. Because I had put my personal self on hold while tending to the marriage, the children, and the career, there were a myriad of left-open wounds I needed to heal and abandoned dreams that I wanted to reweave into my psyche. The image of myself as not-quite-fully present, always one ear to another story, chipped away at my confidence. Here, in this pause, was an opportunity to make some changes.

In 1992, as I turned forty, I left the safety of home to renew myself—moving from central Ohio to New York City—leaving behind four boys with their father. At the time, they were eighteen, sixteen, eleven, and six years old. I rationalized I could become a better mother only if I cared for myself. I was not taught to think like this in my various cultural arenas. My own mother was always completely available to me as a daughter. She did not share stories of other women *who had children,* and who knew anything about this kind of desire to heal. They drank away their cares instead. My girlfriends suggested a vacation. They cited commercials showing active businesswomen cheerfully handing out lunches to children running out the door and then retreating to a Calgon bath in the middle of the afternoon. My family doctor suggested Prozac or Paxil. She was convinced that a few months of drugs would be just the boost I needed to have me back to normal in no time. Only my husband, who up until this point had not participated in the care of the children, was willing to facilitate this growth, realizing the risk and hoping I would choose to return.

Once separated from the responsibility of daily caretaking, what a different life I was having as an academic—with time to organize my own schedule, space to read and think, and plans to eat out instead of cooking for a family of six squeezed between afternoon classes and evening rehearsals. Once away, I no longer experienced myself, daily, as desperately behind, breathless from a lack of sleep, and teary eyed. In my own 450 square foot apartment in the East Village, tiny pleasures made me smile—fragrant soaps, fresh flowers, clean sheets, empty countertops. The space was just as I had left it when I returned. Class assignments were both intriguing to consider and easy to complete. Projects left open on the dining room table waited for me, beckoning me to think, and think again. Living alone—something I had never done—was delightful. I felt highly challenged yet healthy for the first time in years.

People asked me constantly if I wasn't just miserable without the boys. My answer was an embarrassed "no." I loved talking to them on the phone, I anticipated with glee their arrivals when visiting, and I cherished the monthly weekends we spent together, but I was always happy to return to New York to my own apartment where I was flourishing personally.

I am privileged to have had the opportunity to rent a studio apartment in New York while retaining living space in the small college town where I worked and my children had been raised. I am privileged as well to be able to return to graduate school to pick up credentials that would make my career more successful. My married status merged with my class status to increase this privilege, as I was able to expect both the emotional and financial support of my spouse. My profession as a university professor provided the rationale for returning to graduate school, and the cosmology of middle-class, professional, educated adults expected, indeed demanded, that I create opportunities for myself and act on them. It was not the original intention of the second-wave feminist movement to put this demand on white middle-class women without the institutional support that would permit those opportunities to come to fruition, but it was certainly part of the current trend: any privileged woman could have it all without stepping outside the guidelines. Those were the public rules.

My training in feminist theory reminds me to recast the traditional understandings of acts, reverse the roles of male and female to see if the same interpretations remain. It occurs to me that I worked two full-time jobs simultaneously, banking toward that privilege. When a man works two jobs for eighteen years and then is able to lease a luxury car (approximately the same price as the leased apartment over a period of two or three years), the middle-class culture congratulates him for enduring the double life and celebrates the acquisition with him, telling him he deserves it; he worked hard. But when a woman works two jobs and then cashes in, temporarily abandoning one of those jobs in order to enjoy the pleasures of the other, she risks being ostracized—that is, if the job she abandons is mothering. I have come to realize mothering is not cast as a job; it is framed as an identity, and as such it cannot be abandoned.

Both men and women collude in this admonishment: patriarchal as well as soccer-mom common wisdom tell us that choosing any life other than complete subservience to our children is damaging not only to the children but also to the future of our society. If the father were to do this (take time off to increase his career possibilities), it would be read as a sacrifice for the sake of the family. Only the bad mother would voluntarily choose to leave her children behind while pursuing her own dreams. This, instead, is read as selfish and self-centered, and surely damaging to the children.

I am concerned here not with retelling either the worn and familiar tales of midlife crises or of cultural/institutional victimization. I would like, instead, to share a healing story, a story of the renewed relationship made visible by the time away, a story that rarely gets told. This story illustrates that opportunities for growth are provided to both parties—mother and children—when they learn to care for themselves. This is the tale of the youngest child—the child born into the academic-mother/lawyer-father story, the child who never knew life with a stay-at-home mother or a stay-at-home father. Because I am the storyteller, this tale will focus on the mother-child relationship.

LEAVING INSPIRATION:
THE ACT OF BEING CONTAINED
BY THE EXPECTATIONS OF MOTHERING

For the decade preceding this narrative, the mother was on a tenure track at a liberal arts college in Ohio. At the start of that decade, her children were eight, six, one, and not-yet born. She spent days at the university chairing a department, teaching classes, counseling students, and creating and rehearsing pieces for performance. Well buried in her past was a dancer somewhere, and although she was not singly focused on taking her insights to a concert stage, her job at the university allowed her to pursue that interest in the presence of students and colleagues.

It is well documented that the gender of the university professor shapes the experience and the expectations of his or her behavior. Academic men do not have placed on them the same demands as academic women, and they survive in the academic profession of college teaching at a higher rate than their female colleagues because of this. What does it mean to "survive" in the academic sphere? I mean to acquire tenure, to publish adequately, to consult in deep personal ways with students as efficiently as possible, to get promoted quickly, to rank among those earning the highest salaries for the same job. These are the public indicators of success in this profession, and they are achieved more easily by the men. This mother was collapsing from the sheer weight of being everyone's mother.

Meanwhile, the expectations placed on corporate lawyers (the profession of her husband at the time) were, quite simply, to be subservient to a large and unforgiving infrastructure that rewards them mightily for submitting to the corporate demands. Simultaneously those demands remove the lawyers from the family structure with the consolation that providing such a disproportionate income should be enough of a presence. Often neither the corporation nor the participating father sees any problem with this arrangement. The fact that it facilitates the father outstripping the mother in income and therefore promotes the continuation of the father-at-work, mother-at-home dichotomy does not seem to bother anyone. Furthermore, it encourages the mother taking more and more responsibility for the household and the children because her work becomes less and less valuable financially to the family.

The young child in this story, whom we shall call "Alexander," had attended a Montessori preschool. By age five he was so academically precocious that he skipped first grade and moved into second in a new-to-him elite private school that normally holds all children back a year. By the end of third grade, in the mother's two-year absence, he had fallen so far behind that the school counselor was insisting he repeat the grade. The counselor suggested to the mother that "home" for a little boy is wherever his mother is. For two years, she claimed, he had been "away from home, struggling completely on his own." The presence of his father and three older brothers was irrelevant. She insisted a little boy needs to burrow into the soft and receiving shoulder of his loving mother, and only then can he reorganize to face the challenging demands placed on him by the hefty world outside. In the mother's absence, the little boy had had no base of support, and therefore could not thrive academically or emotionally.

INSPIRATION TO GROW:
THE ACT OF USING DANCE-MAKING
AS A TOOL FOR SHARING

The beginning of my story finds little Alex, only six years old when his mother moved to New York, leaving her hundreds of messages on voice mail over a two-year span. During her stay in New York, she transferred these messages to a cassette tape. Upon returning to Ohio, she sat down and worked through them, listening to his reaction to her time away. In response, she proposed they dance together in a March concert she was preparing for. The dance would be about their journeys apart from each other, the frustration of missing each other, the excitement of learning new things, the promise of generosity in the reunion. He seemed to relish in those sessions of creative imaginings, listening to the tape, telling her every detail of what came before and after his messages. He scolded her for not answering him right away. He questioned where she could be at all hours of the day and night. He was, in short, investigating the details of her life without him and revealing the details of his life without her. Merged with moments of running out for fast food together, sifting through his dresser drawers to organize and update his clothes, poring carefully over homework assignments, running after poster board and supplies, those sessions provided for them conversation of days past and vision for days to come.

Together they discarded the messages that were nonsensical out of context, removed the ones that were too personal for anyone else to hear, and commented on the ones they could understand through their emotional thrust even when they could not understand the words. How interesting, they decided, to hear messages without hearing the individual words, how those undiscerned messages let them talk about feelings without worrying about semantics. How expressive he was, and what an attempt he made to manipulate her through his emotional breath! When had she failed him? What did he feel about that? How did it read to hear him give her his phone number, as if he could not count on her knowing it without his cue?

After many hours of scrutiny, they were left with thirty messages that attracted them for various reasons, and they sorted these over and over again. Eventually, she organized them first by time (the computerized voice reminded them of the day, hour, and minute), and then by topic (sleepy mornings, broken shopping promises, school strategies, and the act of telephoning itself). The result was a sound score—a score of little Alex's own voice beckoning to her across the 600 miles, across the psychological distance, across the dependence barrier. A composer then underlaid a solo cello and the mother overlaid a solo dance. This was her gift back to him for leaving.

Text of the Voice Mail Messages
from "Away From Home" (1995)
Choreography and Text: Alex Miller
Dancers: Alex Miller and Gill Wright Miller

Saved. Next message: saved Thursday, February 3rd at 2:47a.m.

My name is Alex Miller. My number is 587-2838 or 0356. But, in your case, in New York it'd be 614-587-2838 or 614-587-0356. But the reason why I called, Mrs. Miller, is: I really have to talk to you. Bye.

(very sleepy voice) Mom? This is Alex . . . on Monday, March seventh. Well, . . . but I wanted to call you. I love you. Now call me back. Call me back. Bye.

Mom? Alex. I just wanted to know if you got the green ninjas. Bye.

Mom? Alex. Uh. I was wondering, uh, if you got the green ninja thing. Call me back. 0356. Bye.

Mom? Alex. I know I'm really up—I'm up really late, but I just want to try to warn you that you told me . . . you told me you'd get the green ninja. . . . Today is Wednesday, the twenty-sixth. . . . Bye.

I take it your beeper's off. . . . I want to know if you got the green ninjas thing. You probably didn't, but I just wanted to know. Bye. Oh wait, call me in the morning. Bye.

Mom? Where are you? It's 9:54, the seventh of February, 1994. And it's Alex and my number is 587-0356. Bye.

You're welcome. Well, so, when might you call me back? Uh-huh? Sure. Well, bye. Bye.

Mom? You must be on the phone. Well, just like I said that one day, when we're at Patty's, we were talking about no more school and but I'd have to do third grade again? Well, I was thinking, like I told you, how 'bout I just don't go to school. . . . I mean, and then you just homeschool me, then I'll go to fourth grade next year. So it's not like no school; it's at home. Call me back. Bye.

Well, Mom, look's like you're on the phone. Today is Thursday; it's 6:54. Bye.

You're just the on-the-phone woman today, aren't you? This is Alex. It's 9:50 p.m., Wednesday the sixteenth, 1994, February. Thank you. Good-bye. –G'bye. –G'bye. –G'bye. –'bye.

Mom, why are you always on the phone? You know who this is. And it's 1:50. Help. It's Alex. Call me back; I'm sleepy. Bye.

Well, you're on the phone. Just call me when you get off. Bye. It's Alex.

Mom, it's about 1:30 in the morning. It's Friday. It's Alex. Call me tomorrow. Call me later on today. Bye.

Mom? Mom? It's the third of March. I just wanted to say good night. It's Alex. Love you. Good night. Bye.

A week before the concert, the mother asked to show the little boy the work she had prepared in his honor, a work she was calling "Away from Home." Reluctantly he came to watch and then announced, "That's my dance, and I need to be in it. You can't dance it by yourself." "I asked you that at the beginning of this process," she scolded. "The concert is this next week. First we'd need to create a duet, and then we'd need to rehearse. There's not time now."

"I can dance already," he said, marginalizing all the years of training she had invested in and asserting intuition alone can design a work. For just an instant, she was transported back to the 1960s and 1970s when the Judson dancers—Yvonne Rainer, Steve Paxton, Trisha Brown, David Gordon, Deborah Hay—were exploring just that.

(I ask the reader now to imagine the cameraperson closing in on the face of a stunned woman, a woman battling with herself, a woman coming to a realization. The camera spirals around from the back of her head: ten feet, five feet, two feet away as the space shifts around, until finally it is directly in front of her, confronting her very right to make a decision at all.) She was tentative, weighing her professional reputation against her responsibilities to her son. Exactly how much control did she need in this relationship, and what was that control all about, all for?

(Cut to the next scene): That evening, he choreographed a nine-minute duet for them and taught it to her within an hour.

(And to the next): They showed his dance to the composer.

"I've seen thousands of dances before," he said, belly-laughing out loud and laying out his credentials as a musician for dance through his snorts. It was an absurd move in front of a nine-year-old.

"You haven't seen this dance before," Alex responded, annihilating the musician's credentials or, rather, decreeing that credentials were not the center of concern here.

In that moment, watching the little boy, she knew this was the line she wanted to step up to. His was the critic she needed to satisfy. It was here that her reputation was being challenged. He was completely uninterested in what some critic might say. She agreed to perform his choreography, and they proceeded like the team of Washington and Hanks in *Philadelphia*. She had a prejudice to overcome and they had a healing to launch and people to convince along the way.

Through this nine-minute dance, "Away from Home," which of the two of them had been away from home is ambiguous. A middle-class mother is "home" when she is with her children. If she moves anywhere else without taking the children, she is away. Because of her university job, she was actually "away" even when she was physically present. Only when they were away on vacation were they "home." A little boy is "home" when he is with his mother. Regardless of where that relationship plays out, if he is with her he is home. However, on the concert stage, where we witness him, he is not at home. This is not a location he frequents, yet there he was touring with her. She shared in his world of the pain of having been separated, and he shared in her world of rehearsing and performing in front of hundreds of people.

The work is about admitting abandonment, and coping with it, through the act of dancing it. It is about the deepening of relations made possible in new and inspiring places. It was about traveling, traveling to these new places, voluntarily and willingly, in spite of trepidation in the journey. This dance work is about the mother and child staying open to meeting each other in these alternative locations—beyond the traditional and single-visioned on-site parenting. It is about *leaving to grow* and about the *inspiration to grow,* and finally about *leaving inspiration* altogether for the experience of merging.

Away from Home

(Opening in a centered pool of light, a small boy with long, soft hair is in a pose, takes another, then a third and fourth. As if announcing his information with his body, he leads rather than responds to the messages.) "Saved," the voice announces, and we wonder if he was. "My name is Alex Miller." *(Change pose.)* "My number is 587-2838, or 0356." *(Change pose again.)* "But, in your case, in New York it'd be 614-587-2838 or 614-587-0356." *(Final change.)* "But the reason I am calling, Mrs. Miller. . . ." A little boy tries to assert himself while contacting his mother who is far away.

(The mother enters while the little boy is watching her from a distance.) "Mom?" the sleepy voice asks. "This is Alex . . . on Monday, March seventh . . . I wanted to call you. I love you. Now call me back." He is still in charge of himself and, he thinks, of her. *(They circle around each other and finally connect.)*

(A soft section of independent moves occurs. She watches from the edges, spinning her hands, lusciously feeling her body sway and curve while he pursues kickboxing and imaginative Ninja Turtle moves. He is in the light; she is not. She attends to him; he attends only to him. His request is at first a command, then a reminder, and finally a frustrating realization that she has probably not done for him what he is asking.) "Oh, wait," he concludes, "call me in the morning" *(as the cello draws out the emotional life of the situation.)* Sad. Isolated. The possibility of abandonment and failure.

(The lights change; the cello picks up.) "Mom? Where are you?" the little voice asks with renewed vigor. *(They dance together, passing each other laterally, tugging at the connecting hand that pulls*

them into and then across each other, barely grasping the opposite hand just before they have traveled too far. Skipping, running, and doing handstands: they play the way a mother and child on a commercial for arthritis medicine might. It is a little too event specific to be spontaneous and a little too free flinging to be real play—more like careful roughhousing.) Meanwhile, he teases her: "So, when might you call me back? Uh-Huh? Sure. Well, good-bye." And then lays out a well-crafted solution for his difficulty in third grade. "Well, I was thinking, like I told you, how 'bout I just don't go to school. . . . I mean, and then you just homeschool me, then I'll go to fourth grade next year." He makes one last try *(as they dance parallel moves, underscoring their similarity.)* "It's not like no school; it's *at home.*"

(Then he runs and runs and runs across the whole space and into her outstretched arms. She spins him around, at first just with his hands, then in a fireman's carry that flings him around to her back, and finally in a tight embrace. The spin winds down and he slides down her body to the floor.)

Another paragraph of telephone commands: "You're just the on-the-phone woman today, aren't you?" followed by, "Why are you always on the phone?" and then a defeated, "Well, you're on the phone. Just call me when you get off. Bye. It's Alex" [in case she didn't know].

(The two dance again, this time climbing over each other. She drags him on her back; he rolls over her; they renegotiate the space. After several exhausting moves, she deposits him in the middle, as the spotlight opens back up. The warmth of the light is juxtaposed against the coolness of the mother leaving him there, alone. He reaches for her with everything he has, but she continues to walk away from him, backward at first, so that she can still see him, then she turns and fades into the unlit space. He reaches still.)

"Mom?" he concludes with a soft, introspective, and gentle voice. "It's the third of March. I just wanted to say good night. It's Alex. Love you. Good night," *(and the spotlight fades to black).*

LEAVING TO GROW:
THE ACT OF DIFFERENTIATING MOTHERING
FROM BEING A MOTHER

It is difficult at best to convey a phenomenological experience in two-dimensional logocentric form. In many ways, it negates the multilayered complex original experience, reducing it to a flat and linear tale. We know of the adage "a picture conveys a thousand words" for still photos. Isadora Duncan, revered forerunner of modern dance, responded to a critic once: "If I could say it, I wouldn't need to dance it." And so, I let the images of the work rest here—his work/our work. However, a few summary remarks of the whole of the experience (leaving, returning, sorting, listening, imagining, creating, scolding, choreographing, performing, and closing) are appropriate. I am conscious of the fact that I work with my own children from my own position of class and race. My expectations both of the experience of mothering and of resisting the institution of mothering come from that stance.

Taking "time out" from a constant, unforgiving, and stressful job has a long and respected history. Mothering is such a job. There is time-honored confusion about mothering—that somehow doing laundry, chauffeuring, and making meals constitutes the bulk of the work, and by engaging in that work, surely children will thrive. Psychologists tell us that the flurry of activity around children makes them feel wanted and valuable, and that providing them with the tools of the subculture they live in allows them to learn what their roles are. For example, if a child is school-aged, the parents (or more often the mother) are expected to create space for studying at home and provide on-site guidance for the completion of these at-home tasks. I am proposing that caring for our children psychologically is not strictly attached to on-site monitoring. On-site monitoring can be imposed by many people, not just a mother.

Furthermore, to ensure the mother is the primary person responsible becomes none other than a monitoring of the mother. When I left the space of our home, I left behind the daily chores of housekeeping, but I never left the daily considerations of my children. To understand the depth of this observation, one needs only to consider whether a child lost through death is forgotten upon no longer attending to his or her daily needs. Of course we realize that the child is forever engraved on the heart of the mother, and if a rendezvous has potential, the elder will care for the relationship actively even in the absence of its daily routines.

Conversely, imposing the separation from the mother's experience and augmenting that separation with the potential for nurturing and growth allows the mother to mend and flourish. She finds herself in a stronger and more able-bodied place to care for the relationships with her children. The heart feeds itself before it feeds the rest of the body. Here, too, the mother must be psychologically healthy and wise to provide adequate care for her offspring. Some mothers can accomplish this in the midst of the daily caretaking. They may have adequate help at home from a partner or an employee. They may have a strong sense of time for themselves from a personality type. Or they may have a lower expectation of what the daily chores involve, functioning easily around piles of laundry, messy living rooms, or multiple repairs that need to be made on the house or the equipment. One other option is to take time out to replenish, repair, or renurture a mother whose needs have not been met.

When we leave our children, whether they are biological offspring, products of our creative imaginations, or projects of great length and intelligence that inspire us deeply, there is a sadness in the parting. However, we provide for ourselves opportunities of distance, perspective, and, most important, renegotiation. Alex and I were strengthened because of the active role we shared in coming back together as a mother with fresh energy and a nine-year-old with newly acquired skills to articulate his own needs.

When we travel apart, we create a distance that allows for panoramic views. Perspective and size become apparent. Large issues and insignificant details come into focus and recede. In this new space, it is possible to tell about oneself and to hear the other's story. Like counting to ten in a heated situation, the months apart gave each of us breath and a new knowledge about and folding into our bodies that provided the internal support we each needed to name our desires and dreams. I was learning to reclaim myself; he was learning to state something for the first time. We both prospered because of this opportunity. Ultimately, this new wakeful state allowed us to renegotiate our relationship. I could let his messy room rest and respect his privacy within that space; he could keep his toys picked up around the public areas of the house. I could enjoy playing tennis with him; he could retreat to his own work in the evening, allowing me space to complete mine. This renegotiation will have a different appearance depending on the age of the child and the needs of the mother, but always there is space for a new consciousness from both parties.

Choosing to reenter a relationship necessarily means redefining both bodies. I am a new person when I return to a familiar place, and the place itself is new as well. I was imagining Alex as a kind of garden, one that I had tilled, planted, and nurtured. It had been growing in my absence and was surely not the same garden when I returned. But a well-cared-for garden, in the absence of the gardener, may be beautifully mature or terribly overgrown in need of pruning and shaping. Perhaps someone else has cared for it, noticing the care that had gone into it before this new gardener stumbled upon it. Or perhaps its very overgrowth introduces the original gardener to a kind of untamed, nearly radical beauty, wild with movement, colors, and aromas circulating with chaotic information. In this case, my leaving made space for his father to learn to care for Alex. The law firm, which had been both a source of personal inspiration and material reward but also a source of escape from the daily tedium of caring for a house and a family, shrank to an appropriate size, and four little boys gained a father.

Had I not left, I would have been unable to continue gardening at all. I was exhausted by the demands of marriage, suburban life in a small college town, and academic glass ceilings. Squeezed between washing last night's dishes, sorting laundry, preparing for class, grading papers, chauffeuring, writing essays, consulting with roof repairmen, preparing dinners, rehearsing dances, and returning phone calls, I knew I had to leave—to care for myself in order to care for them.

Had I not returned, I would have missed the opportunity to develop anew, and in completely new contexts, the relationships I enjoy with my children as precious vessels of friendship, companionship, and activity. I moved into my own house, six blocks away from our family home. The older boys are thriving in Germany, California, and Switzerland. Alex is at home in Ohio living with his father. He stops by my house after school, and I deliver messages from his friends looking for him. He walks my dog; I drop off his forgotten papers at school. I remain highly involved in the energy of his life.

Finally, my children treat me most often as a best friend. Occasionally the more traditional role of mother creeps in, but that is eerily parallel to the role of close friend when one's children are adults. For example, when one of my sons broke off his engagement after a ten-year relationship, he was devastated and collapsed in despair at my house, at my feet. When another of my sons married in June, he and his fiancée called on me daily, with a clear appreciation of my master-organization skills. When little Alex, now tall and sixteen, got his driver's license, we took him out for dinner to go over the so-called contract he had to sign for the privilege of using a family car. And last spring, when the twenty-one-year-old opened in a play in Europe, we flew over to be there for his opening night, skiing afterward, the boys teaching me what to do. These tasks easily replace the cultural expectation of cooking, cleaning, and shopping for appropriate clothing. These tasks—consoling, consulting, and playing together—comprise the role of mentor-friend, helping these young persons grow toward independent adulthood. These are the mothering chores I did not, I will not, give up.

EPILOGUE

Dance, the noun, is a phenomenological event, but so is dance, the verb. Mother, the noun, is also a phenomenological event, as is mother, the verb. They are homonyms; they are not synonyms. Having had children makes one a mother forever, but mothering is an event entirely separate from *being* a mother. When in the presence or absence of our children, our cells carry the memory of the past events, and our present lives are not only enriched but indeed shaped by having had those experiences. Separating ourselves from the dailyness of mothering does not make us no longer a mother; it makes us not presently mothering. Despite patriarchal wisdom, the children will not necessarily suffer, and the mother will have the opportunity to grow into herself and therefore be a better companion to her children. In the most appropriate sense, I am, at this point, a mother without children—but they are surely not children without a mother.

Chapter 11

Perspectives of Substance-Using Women and Human Service Practitioners: Reflections from the Margins

Deborah Rutman
Barbara Field
Suzanne Jackson
Audrey Lundquist
Marilyn Callahan

This chapter is based on original research that examined how policy in Canada deals with the issue of substance use, pregnancy, and mothering, and to identify some alternative ways of addressing this problem that might prove less polarizing and punitive toward women. One focus of this project was to analyze the October 31, 1997, Supreme Court of Canada decision against Ms. G., in which a judge ordered mandatory drug treatment for a young, poor, Aboriginal woman who was addicted to sniffing solvents. Another major component of the project was to uncover the experiences of Aboriginal and non-Aboriginal substance-using pregnant women and mothers, and the practitioners who work most closely with them, in order to explore the impact of existing policies on them and to hear their ideas about approaches that would make or have made a positive difference. This chapter reports our findings in relation to this facet of the project.

SUBSTANCE USE, PREGNANCY, AND MOTHERING

Since the mid-1980s, substance use during pregnancy has been viewed as a significant social problem, prompting increased efforts to

identify mothers who behave in this manner (Gomez, 1977; Ostermann, 1995; Beckett, 1996). In the "Public Policy Statement on
Chemically Dependent Women and Pregnancy" issued by the American Society of Addiction Medicine in 1989, substance use in pregnancy is described as causing "adverse effects on fetal development,"
thus identifying this group of women as "extremely important candi-
dates for intervention and treatment" (as cited in Tanner, 1996,
p. 125). Increasingly, substance use during pregnancy has been equated
with child abuse, and many mothers have lost custody after birth once
their substance use is confirmed. Through the interplay of powerful
discourses, mothers-to-be are transformed into pregnant addicts who
are considered at best sick and at worst criminal. They are identified
as "those bad mothers" who do not adhere to the predominant ideologies of motherhood and as such are caught up in the discursive practices that seek to treat or punish them.

Swift (1995) argues that social intervention is made legitimate
through the creation of categories of scapegoat that indicate deviance
from socially accepted standards. Standards have also been socially
constructed regarding prenatal care for the fetus throughout its gesta-
tional course to maturity. The ideology of good mother/bad mother,
along with the historical doctrine of *parens patriae*—the authority of
the court to make decisions on behalf of those who are unable to do
so—legitimizes intervention in the lives of so-called bad mothers by
the state.

The dichotomous thinking that is reflected in concepts of good and
bad mothers is also replicated in the charged fetus's versus mother's
rights debates. This has led to serious consequences for women in the
United States, where Whiteford and Vitucci suggest that "the war on
drugs has turned into a war on women" (1997, p. 1371). A polarization in the discourse has resulted, pitting mother against child, as the
debate continues around whose rights should be paramount (Boscoe,
1997; Young, 1994; Center for Reproductive Law and Policy, 1996).
Prosecution of women for their behavior during pregnancy has targeted women of color and lower socioeconomic classes; indeed, in
"Florida, South Carolina and in several other states, pregnant women
can also be jailed, purportedly to 'protect the fetus from damage' if
the mother has acknowledged drug use" (Whiteford & Vitucci, 1997,
p. 1372). This research suggests that punitive laws such as these are

less about protecting the unborn and more about punishing women for being poor, pregnant or mothering, and addicted.

As maternal substance use increasingly becomes seen as fetal or child abuse, more pressure is placed on communities to screen pregnant women and report those who are found to be users. Gustavsson and MacEachron (1997) suggest that this policy direction has increased reports to child protection agencies and has resulted in overwhelming workloads for the child protection social workers. "Families are also affected when workloads soar, as resources get directed to completing 'investigations' rather than for providing services to women and their families" (Gustavsson & MacEachron, 1997, p. 679). In the first descriptive study undertaken in Canada, Trocme, McPhee, & Tam (1995) report that in substantiated child abuse cases, substance use in the form of alcohol and drug use is present in 38 percent and 31 percent of cases, respectively.

Besides being ill-resourced to serve families in need, the child protection mandate poses a challenge to dealing effectively with substance-using mothers. Child protection aims to protect children from harm, so it focuses on changing the mother's behavior to conform to the standard that is set out by the worker. However, in addition to operating within compressed time frames, workers have varying amounts of training and understanding of addictions and, therefore, limited ability to assess women's stages of addiction and readiness for change (Callahan, Field, Hubberstey, & Wharf, 1998; Prochaska, Di Clemente, & Norcross, 1992). Assessments also do not always distinguish between patterns of substance use that result in children being neglected or unprotected from abuse, and patterns in which safe arrangements are made when use occurs. The identification of substance use alone becomes proof of child maltreatment.

Although the criminal prosecution model has not been adopted in Canada to punish substance-using pregnant women or mothers, child welfare and mental health legislation has been used in ways that are not incomparable, as the cases of Ms. G. and, more recently, Jeannette Reid illustrate. Both women were impoverished, pregnant, and Aboriginal. Although the state's efforts in Ms. G's case were unsuccessful, Jeannette Reid lost her liberty and custody of her child. In Canada, it can be argued, we punish women primarily through our child protection laws, thus creating barriers to effectively addressing the problem.

Current policy and practice responses shape the experiences of substance-using women and, through these processes, reinscribe their images as deserving of the punitive outcomes ascribed to parents who maltreat their children. Section 13(1) of the British Columbia Child Family and Community Services Act (1994), for example, sets the conditions under which a child is determined to be in need of protection. Once a child is found to need protection from harm that has either occurred or is believed likely to occur, a policy requirement directs a social worker to complete a risk assessment for the particular child and family. The Risk Assessment Model for Child Protection in British Columbia (1996) examines both the possible risks to the safety of the child and those problems and strengths associated with the parents that contribute to or militate against the identified risks. Using this tool, a child may be considered to be at low, medium, or high risk based on a range of additional considerations including the age of the child.

From this assessment the child protection investigator is charged with developing a risk-reduction plan. Substance use by a parent is only one of twenty-three risk factors identified in the assessment tool; however, the severity of the parental alcohol or drug use is ranked on a scale and assigned a number, which then contributes to the child protection worker's understanding of the safety issues for that particular child. As a consequence of the risk-assessment/risk-reduction planning process, the child may be removed from the parent(s) until the child protection worker is satisfied the parent(s) have successfully addressed the substance-use problem. Substance use is frequently featured in current child protection cases, and workers often express frustration with what appear to be low rates of successful amelioration of the problem.

Within the current risk-assessment or risk-reduction frameworks, however, a face-to-face assessment with the substance-using woman is not required to determine her particular use or addiction pattern, motivation toward change, and the type of program that might be most effective to help her. This policy and practice omission in turn contributes to practices in which mothers are directed to programs that may not match their needs. For example, a woman's failure to abstain from substance use following treatment in abstinence-based treatment programs often results in judgments that find the woman unable to safely care for her child. Thus the original assessment of risk becomes compounded further within a perpetuating cycle of pain and failure, in part due to inadequate matching of support, treatment, and individual needs.

RESEARCH PROCESS

This research was undertaken by a group of five women researchers. We were a diverse group, representing Aboriginal and non-Aboriginal backgrounds, academic and nonacademic locations, a mix of ages, incomes, and experience. All of us were mothers and shared a common interest, albeit for a variety of reasons, in the issues related to substance use by pregnant women and mothers.

Our study is based on a thematic analysis of four focus groups with diverse groups of substance-using women, in-depth interviews with three additional women, and three focus groups and three in-depth interviews with Aboriginal and non-Aboriginal human service practitioners who worked with substance-using women and their families.

The first of these focus groups involved seven women who were participating in a pregnancy outreach program specifically geared for women with substance-use problems. Four of these women were pregnant and had other children, two women had recently given birth, and one woman, acting as a support person, was the mother of one of the pregnant women. A second focus group involved women who were clients of the government's child protection ministry. Several of these women's children had been removed by the state. A third focus group was comprised of nine Aboriginal women who had experienced substance-use-related issues, including the removal of their children. These women were participating in an Aboriginal crafts and culture group. A fourth focus group involved six Aboriginal women living on a reserve in northern British Columbia. In addition, we conducted intensive interviews with three other substance-using pregnant women.

To supplement our focus group data, we conducted three focus groups with a diverse group of multidisciplinary practitioners who work with substance-using women. Disciplines represented in the focus groups included addictions counseling, public health nursing, infant development, midwifery, child protection social work, medicine, and hospital social work. Two of the three focus groups involved hospital-based teams/practitioners, and the third involved staff from a community-based needle exchange program. Finally, three in-depth interviews were undertaken. One was with an individual with extensive experience as both a child protection social worker and as an addictions counselor, and two were with Aboriginal drug and alcohol counselors working in an Aboriginal treatment center.

We appreciate the tremendous heterogeneity within the overall population of substance-using pregnant women and mothers. Substance misuse is not a problem that affects just poor women or minority women or younger women—even though these subgroups tend to fit social stereotypes and are probably the most visible and highly targeted groups for intervention services. The women who participated in our study were accessing services from a program based in one of Canada's poorest areas, and more than half of the women were from a visible minority. Thus, we did not have the opportunity to interview middle-class or wealthy, professional women. Consequently, far more diversity undoubtedly exists in the experiences and perspectives of substance-using pregnant women and mothers than our study's findings reflect.

FINDINGS

Context: Women's Experience of Pregnancy, Mothering, and Substance Use

Although it may seem an obvious point, keep in mind that substance-using pregnant women and mothers are women who are addicted to or dependent on substances who then become pregnant, rather than pregnant women who begin to use substances during their pregnancy (see Center for Reproductive Law and Policy, 1996; Noble, 1997). Substance-using pregnant women and mothers do not use substances with the intent of harming their fetuses or children. Instead, they began to use substances well before their pregnancy, have serious drug or alcohol addiction or dependency problems, and then find themselves pregnant or mothering.

In discussing the issue of substance use among pregnant women and mothers, Aboriginal participants reminded us that it should not be analyzed in a vacuum. The systematic dismantling of Aboriginal government and culture has left countless people and multiple generations feeling powerless. The residential school system proved extremely effective in instilling feelings of confusion within the Aboriginal children who attended. In an effort to break down their sense of loyalty to their family, the residential school ridiculed and rejected their whole way of life and the source of their cultural pride and self-identity. This system also forced the children to reject everything that they had ever believed themselves to be. Generations of children were removed from their parents and communities. The residential school, acting as an agent for the colonial system, taught these children to hate their parents, themselves, and their culture. The effects of these teachings have spilled over onto the self-esteem and self-confidence of every generation since. The horrific abuses that these children experienced left many hollow shells or shells full of rage.

As is the nature of substance use, what started as occasional use of drugs or alcohol to minimize psychological pain soon turned into a raging epidemic among numerous First Nations people who attended residential schools as well as in all subsequent generations. Although First Nations people have come a long way in reclaiming their birthright, cultural pride, and practices, the feelings of powerlessness and the problems of low self-esteem and substance dependence are still very much alive. Participants emphasized that much of Aboriginal people's destructive and self-destructive behavior—and in particular their substance use—can be linked to residential schools:

> At the residential school, they did our thinking for us. They took away our culture, our language, our parents, our guidance. My mom didn't teach me. When I grew up, I followed my mom. I couldn't teach my children. All I could give was my love. That hurt so much—that I lost all that through the silly residential school [crying]. When I left the residential school, I thought I was so smart. Yet at eighteen I didn't even know I could get pregnant, or that I was pregnant. So, many of our people thought that alcohol was how to get to know people. That's what I got into. I drank for all of my life except when I was in jail.

In addition, Aboriginal and non-Aboriginal women alike emphasized that some women may not know they are pregnant until some months into their pregnancy; others may not learn of the potential damage that their substance use may cause until late in their pregnancies.

> I did quite a bit of rock. Then I found out I was two months pregnant. I didn't realize it 'til then.

Many participants in our focus groups spoke of their tremendous, relentless feelings of guilt and shame regarding their substance use during pregnancy. For some, it led to suicidal thoughts and feelings of utter despair:

> When I was pregnant, I felt trapped by my feelings of guilt. I was in my eighth month when I came here [to the pregnancy outreach program]. It was then that I read this paper how my baby could be affected, what kinds of damage there could be—I felt so bad, so guilty. I wanted to kill myself.

However, as has been reported in the literature (Tanner, 1996; Bruce & Williams, 1994), participants noted that for them, pregnancy and motherhood presented themselves as windows of opportunity to try to turn things around, to address their substance-use problems, in order to help their children have the healthiest possible start in life.

> Me and the baby went through withdrawal. I still do cigarette smoking. I know it's not healthy, but it's better than doing rocks. I'm finally away from it. I'm happy . . . I understand rehab situations. I want to give the baby a fighting chance.

Moreover, for our participants, women's motivation during pregnancy to quit or reduce their substance use was prompted not only by their wish to promote their fetuses' health, but also by their strong desire to keep their babies after birth:

> My old man and me, we've been doing prenatal, parenting . . . All to make sure we can keep the baby.

> I don't want the baby caught up in the system. He seems healthy and active so far. I have had three kids prior to this that I never had.

Women's deep desire to mother their babies and not have them apprehended by the state seems to be conspicuously overlooked and rendered invisible within most of the literature and media coverage concerning substance-using pregnant women and mothers. Indeed, the impression that the public is given is that "these women" care about neither their fetuses' or children's health nor about their own mothering responsibilities; they are said to "relinquish" their children—presumably because of lack of interest in them—and to have little desire to remain in contact with them. The picture that emerges through discussions with substance-using women is very different, however. Through our focus groups and interviews, we were privileged to hear from women about their feelings, and we learned that the depiction of women as oblivious and unfeeling is both inaccurate and unjust. Women's connections to their children are strong and deep. Many women will try to do whatever they can—or have been told to do by authorities—in order to maintain hope that they will keep their children.

Ideological Context to Policy and Practice: Construction of Substance-Using Women As Bad Mothers

A central theme and starting point in human service professionals' discussion of existing policy and practice was the philosophical underpinnings of policy and how ideologies have affected the types of services and resources available, as well as practitioners' approaches to working with substance-using women.

A primary facet of current dominant ideologies is their dichotomous nature. Dichotomous thinking, by definition, frames an issue in an either/or fashion; with this issue, dichotomous framing leads to the pitting of a woman's interests against those of her fetus or child(ren). For example, one informant who had extensive experience as an addictions counselor and a child protection worker noted that dichotomous thinking was predominant in the child welfare field and was demonstrated when professional concern was directed at either a mother's health or the (unborn) child's health, and when a woman's rights and best interests were pitted against those of her fetus or child.

One of the most deeply entrenched set of dichotomous assumptions and beliefs, evident in child welfare policy and prevalent among many practitioners, concerns the idea that mothers who use substances are not, and perhaps cannot be, safe or good mothers (Boyd, 1999). These assumptions have greatly influenced current child protection policies, risk-assessment protocols, and the practice of multidisciplinary family health professionals. For example, one practitioner spoke of how this ideology had so influenced child protection social workers' decisions regarding whether a substance-using mother could care for her child(ren) safely that the decision-making process became, in effect, formulaic:

The question [becomes]: "Is a woman using? Isn't she using?" Oh, she's using. She must go to treatment now. She doesn't go to treatment, she doesn't get her baby. And it's like this, kind of . . . a built in formula.

Substance-using women also recognized that, having been constructed to be bad mothers, their interactions with their children would be seen to reveal their maternal disinterest or inadequacy. The disjunction between this construction and women's own experiences and perspectives was quite striking. For instance, participants emphasized that when they did not attend case conferences or visit children who had been apprehended, it was not due to disinterest but because of their own feelings of shame and guilt about their addiction problems:

My son isn't in my care. Even though I've been here [at the pregnancy outreach program] since my eighth month of pregnancy, they took him away. I don't see him very much. It's too hard . . .

I wrote a letter to my dad [to give to my children] when I was in treatment, that their mommy's in a recovery house and the she's getting better and she loves them with all her heart. And that we're going to be together again. But while I was in there I didn't think I could face anybody, and I didn't think I could look at them and say, "I'm an addict and I'm trying to smarten up."

Predominance of an Abstinence Model

An abstinence model for the treatment of addictions—currently the predominant model in British Columbia—was similarly described by participants as being dichotomous in that it was all or none, black or white, and assumed and required that people with substance dependencies could just say no. Anything less than this could be considered personal failure. Indeed, our informants suggested that an abstinence model had shaped the biases and expectations of practitioners, thus creating a lens through which all progress was monitored. These expectations, or "magical thinking" as one informant referred to them, also often led to a pass or fail, shame-based mentality on the part of both the workers and the women they are trying to assist. The limits of this approach for marginalized women with complex multiple problems, whose addictions may have spanned twenty years or more, were clearly expressed by practitioners, as the following comment indicates:

If abstinence is the only outcome you can see as a sign of success, then of course you are going to see everybody as noncompliant, resistant, and in denial. Because not everybody can do that in the time we can have with them.

The historic treatment model from which many programs and policies had developed was based on research findings with white, middle-class males. Although an abstinence approach may have been effective with men, our informants suggested that those techniques are not generalizable to a multiethnic, polydrug-using group of pregnant women and mothers.

The Pitting of Woman versus Fetus/Child and Family-Focused versus Child-Focused Practice

In discussing existing ideology, policies, and practice, participants also observed that policymakers and practitioners continued to engage in dichotomous thinking in relation to child-focused versus family-focused practice. This policy debate must be flagged, both because dichotomous thinking arguably runs counter to both a family health approach and to woman-centered treatment models, and because it has influenced the practice of many professionals who work with substance-using mothers:

I think you have conflicts because we from the pediatric community point of view have a very child-focused approach . . . And I think that some of colleagues that we interact with bring a more family-focused approach, a parent-focused approach. It does inevitably mean occasional disagreement when you are kind of more batting for the mom in the family than maybe you are for the baby . . .

This longstanding issue has plagued the child welfare field for decades and has resulted in pendulum-like swings in policy and program development. Although many observers and workers within the child welfare system have been highly critical of such divisive, either/or thinking—arguing instead that good, holistic, family-focused practice will fundamentally benefit children as well—overall, dichotomous thinking seems firmly entrenched. Currently, largely as a result of the 1995 Gove Inquiry, BC child welfare policy emphasizes the "paramountcy" of the child. This swing toward child-focused practice also has been fanned by the media's and the public's scrutiny and ongoing criticism of the Ministry for Children and Family Development. Participants observed that, as a consequence of such intense public and government scrutiny, the Ministry's message to front-line child protection social workers was that they would be held personally accountable for removal decisions and their outcomes. As a result:

> [Ministry social workers] are coming in with no alternatives, and they are under the gun right now. They are scared out of their minds that they are going to lose their jobs. And so they are coming up with the most cautious approach that they can think of. Which is removal. Which is probably the worst possible time to remove the baby, at birth.

Practitioners in our study were sympathetic to the issues and pressures facing these social workers. However, participants' comments indicated that they believed that this policy direction, by instilling fear and "cover your ass" thinking within workers, had serious, negative ramifications for practitioners as well as families. Moreover, participants were most concerned about the negative impacts for families of the policy direction to remove children in keeping with this "most cautious approach," especially when removal came at birth.

Stereotyping, Homogenizing, and Ghettoizing Women Who Use Substances

Finally, in discussing dominant ideologies and their impact on policy and practice, participants spoke about the public's—and professionals'—tendency to ghettoize women with substance-use problems:

> . . . and I agree that it has got to be across the community, not ghettoizing, which was our great fear. That the minute we start talking about substance-using women, in people's mind's eye, it's a ghettoized population there. And it isn't.

As participants pointed out, ghettoizing women with substance dependency/addiction issues turns them into an homogeneous group of, presumably, indigent, welfare-dependent, possibly homeless, marginalized, and, more than likely, Aboriginal women. Ghettoizing renders women's individuality and their unique circumstances, experiences, and needs invisible. Moreover, ghettoizing can lead to professionals limiting and focusing their outreach efforts on those women whom they expect will fit prevailing racist and classist stereotypes of substance-using pregnant women or mothers. It becomes in effect a self-fulfilling prophecy as certain groups become overrepresented in the affected and targeted population:

> First Nations people and women are disproportionately criminalized for their drug use. If you are a lawyer who has a regular heroin habit in Kitsilano, how likely is it that you are going to come under the scrutiny of the state?

Unbecoming Mothers: Substance-Using Women's Experience of State Intervention

Substance-using women are acutely aware that many professionals hold negative and prejudiced views toward them because they are pregnant or mothering. As noted previously, many women already experience tremendous feelings of guilt and shame about their substance use during pregnancy. However, these feelings are often fueled by the women's perception that workers, mirroring societal attitudes, are shaming and blaming—that workers assume that the women, because they are addicts, are both deceitful and unfit, uncaring, and even abusive as mothers. One woman told of an experience involving a social worker who brought the police with her when making a home visit to see the woman's baby:

> But one social worker, she brought some cops to my place. It was like a drug raid. They wanted to see the baby. She was fine; she was sleeping.

According to Aboriginal participants, another facet of practitioners' prejudice was their racism. For example, one Aboriginal woman believed that her physician accused her of abusing her infant because of the doctor's prejudicial beliefs about Native, substance-using women; the physician was not aware of a particular type of physical occurrence in some Aboriginal infants and instead was quick to label the markings as signs of abuse.

> My doctor said I was abusing my baby because of Mongolian spots. She said there were marks on his back that looked like abuse. But if you're Aboriginal or Asian, you know that they're just Mongolian spots and that the spots go away.

First Nations people also clearly expressed anguish over the removal of their children as a result of their substance use, especially when the child went to live in non-Aboriginal homes:

> The white man took my kids away—all my kids. I could give them love, but not change their diapers. I think they should be brought up in traditional homes.

Women's distress about practitioners' blaming and prejudicial attitudes was heightened by their recognition of the power that certain professionals held, particularly in relation to child protection/apprehension issues. Participants expressed that they generally felt powerless in their interactions with medical and child welfare authorities. Moreover, their feelings of powerlessness were exacerbated by their belief that practitioners' prejudicial attitudes prevented them from seeing women as individuals or from acknowledging women's efforts toward recovery. As one focus group participant shared with us:

> Here's a story: I love my husband. When I was in the hospital with my last baby, I was so happy to see my husband. I mean, I really wake up in the morning, and there he is, with his morning breath and all, and I can just say, "Babe, I love you!" But when I was in the hospital, there was one nurse who said that he was giving me drugs. Like, that's why I was happy to see him, because he was giving me drugs. I felt like that one nurse, she had so much power . . .

Overall, the impact of women's experience of practitioners' prejudice and their sense of powerlessness was a deep fear and distrust of many professionals. Women's fears were palpable, ever-present, and borne from troubled and demoralizing experiences. Their fears also had a specific focus: that their babies would be removed by child welfare authorities. Moreover, their fears seemed heightened by their recognition of the Ministry for Children and Family Development's current policy to earmark maternal substance use as a high-risk factor, one that often contributed to child protection investigations, risk assessment, and apprehension orders. One woman described her anxiety regarding what she believed to be her doctor's power to apprehend her baby:

> Some people are so prejudiced. For example, the doctor at the hospital. She didn't like me. [I still worry] that she's going to find some way to take my baby away.

As has been found in the literature, women's distrust and fear could result in their avoidance of alcohol and drug treatment and/or perinatal care (Goldberg, 1995; Metsch et al., 1995; Noble, 1997). One focus group participant spoke to this point by vowing to travel to another province to deliver her baby, in order to help ensure that authorities would not apprehend her child on the basis of what she deemed prejudice (as, in her opinion, had happened before).

> [Crying] I will leave BC to have this baby. I'm so scared. My apartment is fine. I even have furniture. But I'm so scared that they're going to take away my baby. I've been through this before. I was clean for four months. But they still took my baby. I had her for two days before the bailiffs came in to take her away.

In addition, from participants' perspectives, the predominant abstinence model does not recognize the realities of people's lives, including why people use substances, what other issues people are contending with, and what purposes substance use might serve. An abstinence model also does not recognize that recovery and healing are processes that take considerable time and tremendous effort, most often involve relapses and backslides, and are best measured in very small steps. Substance-using women strongly emphasize that women's every step toward recovery, however small, needs to be appreciated. When this does not happen, women feel demoralized and unsupported. This can constitute a real barrier to accessing treatment, as our participants shared with us:

> I was trying, even at that late date, to do something. And they didn't listen. . . . But now, I have a beautiful apartment. And I have food!!! I have coffee and tea and sugar and milk in the fridge! And soap. People overlook that. But if people could see that. It's those stupid little things like that, that mean a lot.

Women need to have the space to voice their sense of their progress and setbacks, and those working with women need to be especially attuned to the significance that these milestones, however small, might hold. Clearly, pregnant women's avoidance of addictions treatment or prenatal care is a potentially disastrous consequence of current practice and policy. This unintended outcome, ironically, can result in significant harm or neglect to both women and children.

Along these lines, substance-using women spoke emphatically about how their worries regarding their babies' possible apprehension, apparently instilled or reinforced through scare tactics by some professionals, had the adverse effect of heightening their addiction problems:

> I'm so scared they're going to take my baby away. . . . They think that'll make me better. But what they do is making me a worse addict.

An even more direct connection between actually losing their children and abusing substances was made by women whose children had been apprehended by the state. Women spoke plainly that for them, after their child(ren) were removed, there was little reason to remain clean and sober:

> After they took my baby away, I was on the phone with my dealer in half an hour. I have to keep remembering how happy I was before I was addicted, when I was in control of my own life. . . . After I lost my kids, I thought: "Who the hell cares?"

The women's point was clear: why would they bother staying clean when that which they cared about most—their children—was gone for them? In view of women's experiences, their sense of hopelessness and the self-destructive behaviors that could stem from their feelings of futility were understandable. Women's experiences also have clear implications both about the effects of existing policies/approaches and in terms of directions for alternatives: For substance-using pregnant women, using threats, fear, or intimation that child(ren) will be apprehended if mothers continue to use is a major barrier to women's recovery. Fear heightens women's addiction problems. Alternatively, having the hope of keeping their children is a major motivator for women to quit/reduce. As one woman told us, speaking to the importance of instilling hope:

> G.'s my favorite nurse. There was this one time, and I screwed up, and I got really scared—what would this mean for the baby? But G. said, "Don't feel guilty. Your baby's active." That's the kind of people we need. When I come down, it's people like G. I have to talk to. . . . Before I got here, I wanted to kill myself.

DISCUSSION: DIRECTIONS FROM WOMEN AND HUMAN SERVICE PRACTITIONERS

Paradigm Shifts

According to our project's informants, a primary starting point in identifying or envisioning policy and practice responses is the philosophical and value base of policies and practices. Substance-using women, Aboriginal women, and human service practitioners clearly and emphatically spoke of the need for a fundamental shift in the ideologies and societal attitudes relating to pregnant women's and mothers' substance use. Most important, ideologies and attitudes need to shift away from their dichotomous framing of the problem and solution, to a more holistic and humanistic conceptualization.

A nondichotomous framing of the issues is exemplified by a harm-reduction approach to working with substance-using pregnant women. Many participants spoke about the importance of shifting to a harm-reduction philosophy and of its positive consequences in practice. As this practitioner told us:

> I think what [the worker] did differently was [that] the expectations from the beginning weren't so rigid. She never presented to the mom: This, this, and this. It was just, "I'm worried about you. You are having another baby. You are having trouble taking care of the one you have, you know. What can we do?" It wasn't putting such a burden on her that she had to commit for a lifetime process.

Another ideological shift that reflects a nondichotomous framing of the issues relates to the place of child welfare practitioners in the treatment of substance-using, pregnant women and mothers. Child welfare workers need to be part of a supportive, pregnancy outreach team for substance-using women. Clearly, however, child welfare workers' mere presence on this team is not sufficient; they must be working from the same harm-reduction, woman-focused philosophical base and be as knowledgeable in the area of women's addictions as their colleagues. Moreover, it must be evident that the intent and goal of having child welfare practitioners present in women's treatment is to augment women's feelings of power and control over the situation, rather than the reverse:

[I]f she is going to be involved anyway, let's get her, the social worker, involved prior to the last minute. Help the woman turn the tables from being frightened of seeing the social worker and not feeling she has any power. Being able to say to her, "You work for the government. I am going to need your help."...So that they are not the victim of, they are actually being able to ask the government, saying, "I want to keep this baby and this is what I want you to do to help me do that."

Another ideological shift that would reflect nondichotomous framing is evident in the values underpinning Scottish child welfare policy. In Scotland, a child's apprehension by the state is viewed as a failure of the child welfare system, rather than a failure of an individual mother or family. This philosophical base implies that the state is obligated to try to support the parents in every way possible; implicit as well is the notion that providing support to the parent(s) is the best means of supporting the child and that the parents' and child's interests are linked rather than opposed to each other. Another key implication of this philosophy is that the state has a responsibility in supporting the woman in order to support the child.

Participants felt strongly that adoption of the Scottish model in child welfare would have positive consequences for substance-using women and their children. At the same time, they emphasized that such an ideological shift would be dramatic, given current trends in Canadian child welfare policy:

[I]n Scotland, [the] removal of a child from a family is seen as a failure of the system. Starting from there would be a qualitative shift from our current practice. And it's almost, how do we move to that place, where we have done everything that we could to support that mother/child pair? And that if that has to be broken down, then we also look at that critically to say how have we failed? What else could we have done? Knowing that sometimes, of course, it will have to happen, but it better be a last resort, rather than what's becoming a first resort out of fear.

As was discussed in our case study, community awareness and education were seen as key prevention strategies. Participants believed that children and youth needed to be informed about the effects of maternal substance abuse, fetal alcohol syndrome/effects (FAS/E), and about reproductive health and birth control. Participants also emphasized the importance of openly discussing the causes of (maternal) substance use (particularly within an Aboriginal context). It was hoped and presumed that open community discussion would promote the destigmatization of people with addiction problems, and would lead to community action and support for substance-using women.

[T]he better method is to educate our young people from the start about the long-term effects of FAS. You have to think in terms of the seventh generation. Each of us takes our personal cycle; we're the start of the intervention.

Effective Treatment Approaches: What Works, from Women's Perspective

In addition to needed philosophical or ideological shifts, participants identified a number of key dimensions of effective treatment approaches. These were

- Treatment programs geared specifically for pregnant women
- Programs/facilities for aftercare
- Holistic care
- Outreach
- Residential facility with homelike environment
- Peer support/counseling; group work
- Nonjudgmental attitudes of practitioners, unconditional support
- Individualized treatment plans made collaboratively with women

There is a pressing need for treatment programs geared for pregnant women and mothers. Women spoke of their need for safety, support, and understanding in a nonthreatening environment; they also spoke of the importance of being with other pregnant women and mothers who had gone through comparable experiences. As an extension, participants spoke of the tremendous importance of aftercare; programs and facilities need to be available to women who are seeking support with mothering and other issues.

Effective treatment for pregnant women and mothers is holistic and aims to address and support a woman in all domains of her life, including her health, housing, social, and spiritual needs. Several participants observed that women's social needs were frequently ignored in existing treatment programs, even though loneliness and social isolation often contributed to their substance use. In addition, ongoing, supportive outreach is a critical component of effective care. Numerous participants spoke of the importance of having someone "come looking for you" in order to demonstrate caring and concern, and to provide the message that "you matter" to them. Participants also noted that substance-addicted women with low self-esteem found it difficult to believe that anyone would care; thus, outreach needs to be both persistent yet nonjudgmental, and it should meet a woman on her own terms. As well, peer support is a critical dimension of effective care. Many women spoke of their desire to help others overcome their addiction problems as soon as they themselves had progressed further in their recovery. Peer support and mentoring were discussed at length as a means to facilitate healing even after a person's participation in a formal treatment program had ended.

Substance-using pregnant women and mothers need the unconditional support and compassion of practitioners and peer counselors. Unconditional support means that women will be "given the benefit of the doubt," that their relapses or "screwups" are not judged, and that their day-to-day accomplishments, however seemingly modest, are celebrated. Unconditional support also instills in people a sense of hope, which has been shown to be a major factor that turns things around for women with addictions problems (White, 1998).

A final dimension of effective treatment is the way in which practitioners work with women to set treatment goals and plans. Plans made collaboratively with women, with goals set by women themselves in recognition of their unique circumstances and needs, are apt to be most effective. A collaborative approach signifies respect for the woman, appreciates her individuality, and empowers her in her relationships with others.

Healing Through Cultural Renewal: What Works, from Aboriginal Women's Perspective

Finally, Aboriginal women spoke of the tremendous importance of cultural (re)connection as a means to facilitate healing and support recovery. Native treatment centers, especially those designed for women, were seen as one valuable means to connect women with traditional culture:

> The Recovery House really helped me a lot. It's all First Nations women there. Being there taught me how to have and be a friend. How to respect people. How to teach and ask other people to respect my boundaries.

Why don't they put more native treatment centers all over Canada? They help. They really help!

Another means to help pregnant women and mothers with serious substance-use problems that was identified by participants was through intensive, round-the-clock support and, if necessary, supervision, focusing on women's connection with culture. This might come about through taking a woman into one's home, accompanying her on errands and activities, all the while attempting to reinstill in her a sense of respect, confidence, and pride, and emphasizing that she and her fetus are valued within the community:

When I was drinking, this family noticed me. They saw I was homeless. They took me into their home. They wouldn't let me into town alone. I never went anywhere unchaperoned. I ended up going with that man's son and having his child—we have a hereditary princess. I went into AA [Alcoholics Anonymous] when I was eight months' pregnant. That was a good experience. I wouldn't have chosen it, but it snuck up on me. . . . Now I don't hang out with drinkers. I do a lot of ceremonies. Sweats. That's my way of being clean and sober.

At the same time, participants spoke to the significance of cultural reconnection programs and activities that did not necessarily have a treatment focus; these activities promoted healing through the teaching and practice of traditional ways. For many Aboriginal people, (re)connection with traditional culture is instrumental to healing, as it instills and/or restores feelings of self-respect, pride, and identity that may have been all but extinguished. The following comments by participants speak to the overwhelming value of reconnection with culture and tradition for Aboriginal women, many of whom had successfully addressed their substance addiction:

I used to think I was a terrible addict. Now I say to myself, "Wow, you can sew moccasins!"

Grandma M. was teaching this class, making moccasins and trinkets. I feel really proud of myself, that I can say I make things. I can go to powwows and say, "I made these myself." I tell everyone I know, "There's a class where you can learn things like this." It does so much for you and for your kids. They're learning and don't even know it. I'm so proud of my daughter. We just went to a powwow and she danced, and spoke with a microphone to over 600 people. . . . I've been really involved with my daughter's school. . . . The teacher asked me about traditional teachings that I had learned. I talked for one hour. I was so proud to be answering those questions. I didn't think that I knew that much.

[I]t's really beneficial for the kids to be exposed to those kinds of cultural things. Because growing up without identity really hurts. It took me until I was twenty-five years old to realize that, to be proud that I can talk the Okanagan language, that I know canning . . .

As is evident from these comments, as well as being a key to recovery, connecting with traditional culture can help prevent substance use among Aboriginal people, especially youths. In discussing their participation in cultural activities, participants spoke of their role as learners and also as teachers with younger generations. Many participants viewed their culture as a source of tremendous strength and as a means to instill pride in young people, which in turn could serve to insulate youth from the pressures and challenges that lead many to substance use and addiction.

REFERENCES

Beckett, K. (1996). Fetal rights and "crack moms": Pregnant women in the war on drugs. *Contemporary Drug Problems, 22,* 587-612.

Boscoe, M. (1997). Compulsory treatment orders for pregnant women. Electronic mailing list: Policy Action Research List, posted March 17, 1997. Women's Health Clinic <womenshealthclinic.org>.

Boyd, S. (1999). *Mothers and illicit drugs: Transcending the myths.* Toronto, ON: University of Toronto Press.

British Columbia Child, Family and Community Services Act. (1994). Victoria, BC: Queen's Printer.

Bruce, L. & Williams, K. (1994). Drug abuse in pregnancy. *Journal of the Society of Obstetricians and Gynaecologists of Canada, 24,* 1469-1476.

Callahan, M., Field, B., Hubberstey, C., & Wharf, B. (1998). *Best practices in child welfare.* Child, Family and Community Research Program, University of Victoria, Victoria, BC.

Center for Reproductive Law and Policy. (1996). *Punishing women for their behaviour during pregnancy: An approach that undermines women's health and children's interests.* New York: Author.

Goldberg, M. (1995). Substance-abusing women: False stereotypes and real needs. *Social Work, 40*(6), 789-798.

Gomez, L. (1997). *Misconceiving mothers: Legislators, prosecutors and the politics of prenatal drug exposure.* Philadelphia: Temple University Press.

Gustavsson, N. & MacEachron, A. (1997). Criminalizing women's behavior. *The Journal of Drug Issues, 27*(3), 673-687.

Metsch, L., Rivers, J., Miller, M., Bohes, R., McCoy, C., Morrow, C., Bandstra, E., Jackson, V., & Gissen, M. (1995). Implementation of a family-centered treatment program for substance abusing women and their children: Barriers and resolutions. *Journal of Psychoactive Drugs, 27*(1), 73-78.

Noble, A. (1997). Is prenatal drug use child abuse? Reporting practices and coerced treatment in California. In P. Erikson, D. Riley, Y. Cheung, & P. O'Hare (Eds.), *Harm reduction: A new program for drug policies and programs* (pp. 174-194). Toronto, ON: University of Toronto Press.

Ostermann, S. (1995). A history of treatment for chemically dependent women. *Focus,* September, 5-6.

Prochaska, J., Di Clemente, C., & Norcross, J. (1992). In search of how people change: Applications to addictive behaviour. *American Psychologist, 47*(9), 1102-1114.

Report of the Royal Commission on Aboriginal Peoples. (1996). Ottawa, ON: Queen's Printer.

The Risk Assessment Model for Child Protection in British Columbia. (1996). British Columbia Ministry for Children and Families, Child Protection Consultation Services. Victoria, BC: Queen's Printer.

Sterling-Collins, R. (1991). Indian policies: Historical to present day perspective. Unpublished paper. University of Victoria, Victoria, BC.

Swift, K. (1995). *Manufacturing bad mothers: A critical perspective on child neglect.* Toronto, ON: University of Toronto Press.

Tanner, L. (1996). *The mother's survival guide to recovery: All about alcohol, drugs and babies.* Oakland, CA: New Harbinger Publications.

Trocme, N., McPhee, D., & Tam, K. (1995). Child abuse and neglect in Ontario: Incidence and characteristics. *Child Welfare, 74*(3), 563-586.

White, S. (1998). *How professional systems instruct mothers recovering from substance misuse.* Unpublished master's thesis, University of Victoria, Victoria, BC.

Whiteford, L. & Vitucci, J. (1997). Pregnancy and addiction: Translating research into practice. *Social Science Medicine, 44*(9), 1371-1380.

Young, I. (1994). Punishment, treatment, empowerment: Three approaches to policy for pregnant addicts. *Feminist Studies, 20*(1), 33-57.

Index

Order a copy of this book with this form or online at:
http://www.haworthpress.com/store/product.asp?sku=5177

UNBECOMING MOTHERS
The Social Production of Maternal Absence

_____in hardbound at $39.95 (ISBN: 0-7890-2452-7)

_____in softbound at $29.95 (ISBN: 0-7890-2453-5)

Or order online and use special offer code HEC25 in the shopping cart.

COST OF BOOKS_____

POSTAGE & HANDLING_____
(US: $4.00 for first book & $1.50
for each additional book)
(Outside US: $5.00 for first book
& $2.00 for each additional book)

SUBTOTAL_____

IN CANADA: ADD 7% GST_____

STATE TAX_____
(NJ, NY, OH, MN, CA, IL, IN, PA, & SD
residents, add appropriate local sales tax)

FINAL TOTAL_____
(If paying in Canadian funds,
convert using the current
exchange rate, UNESCO
coupons welcome)

☐ **BILL ME LATER:** (Bill-me option is good on
    US/Canada/Mexico orders only; not good to
    jobbers, wholesalers, or subscription agencies.)
☐ Check here if billing address is different from
    shipping address and attach purchase order and
    billing address information.

Signature_____

☐ **PAYMENT ENCLOSED: $**_____

☐ **PLEASE CHARGE TO MY CREDIT CARD.**

☐ Visa ☐ MasterCard ☐ AmEx ☐ Discover
☐ Diner's Club ☐ Eurocard ☐ JCB

Account # _____

Exp. Date_____

Signature_____

Prices in US dollars and subject to change without notice.

NAME_____

INSTITUTION_____

ADDRESS_____

CITY_____

STATE/ZIP_____

COUNTRY_____ COUNTY (NY residents only)_____

TEL_____ FAX_____

E-MAIL_____

May we use your e-mail address for confirmations and other types of information? ☐ Yes ☐ No
We appreciate receiving your e-mail address and fax number. Haworth would like to e-mail or fax special
discount offers to you, as a preferred customer. **We will never share, rent, or exchange your e-mail address
or fax number.** We regard such actions as an invasion of your privacy.

Order From Your Local Bookstore or Directly From
The Haworth Press, Inc.
10 Alice Street, Binghamton, New York 13904-1580 • USA
TELEPHONE: 1-800-HAWORTH (1-800-429-6784) / Outside US/Canada: (607) 722-5857
FAX: 1-800-895-0582 / Outside US/Canada: (607) 771-0012
E-mailto: orders@haworthpress.com

For orders outside US and Canada, you may wish to order through your local
sales representative, distributor, or bookseller.
For information, see http://haworthpress.com/distributors

(Discounts are available for individual orders in US and Canada only, not booksellers/distributors.)
PLEASE PHOTOCOPY THIS FORM FOR YOUR PERSONAL USE.
http://www.HaworthPress.com   BOF04